THE ULTIMATE PEGAN DIET COOKBOOK

Tasty Quick and Simple Pegan Diet Recipes Merging the Best of Paleo and Vegan Diets for Lifelong Wellness

DR. RYAN BERGER

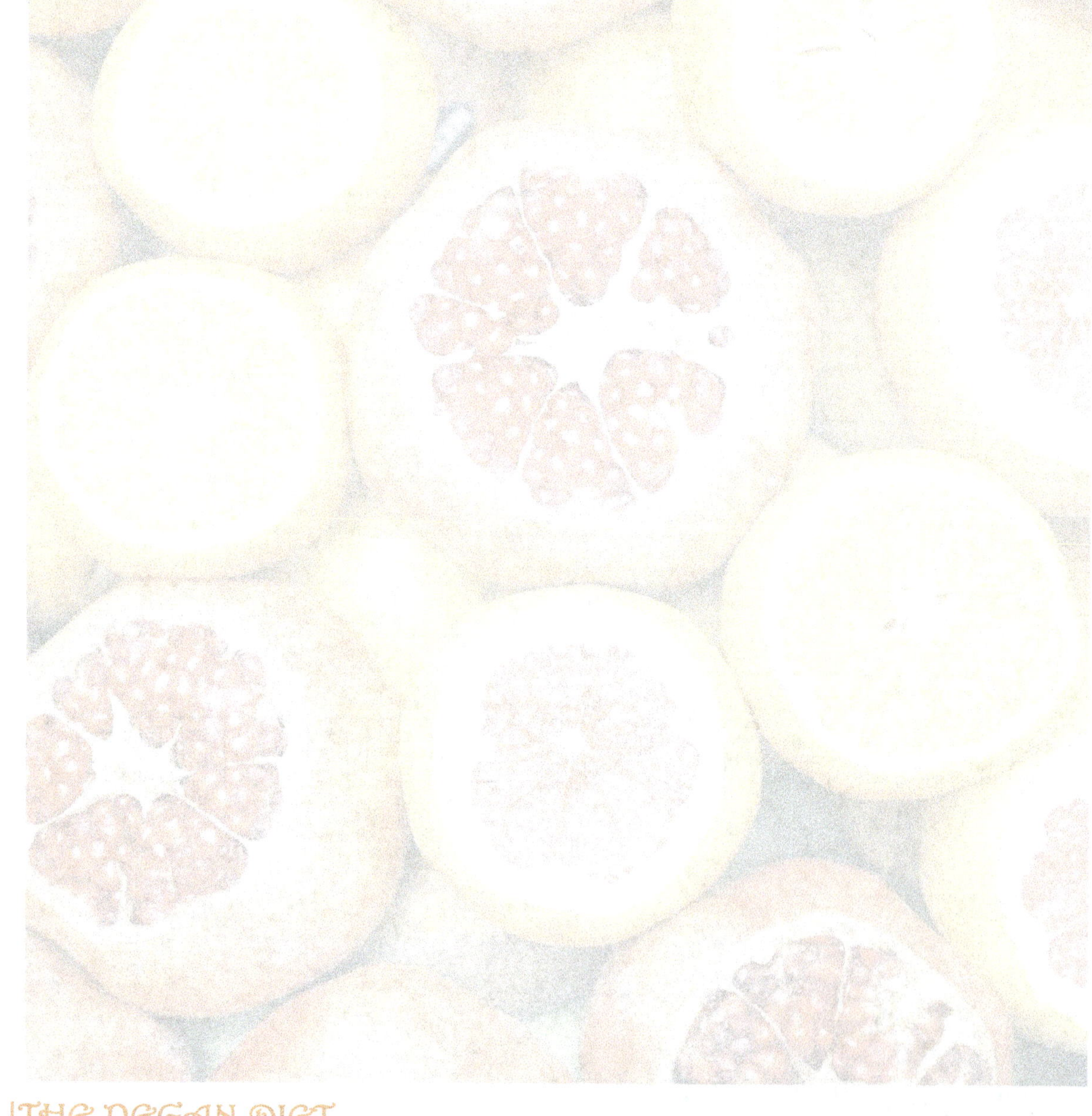

Table of Contents

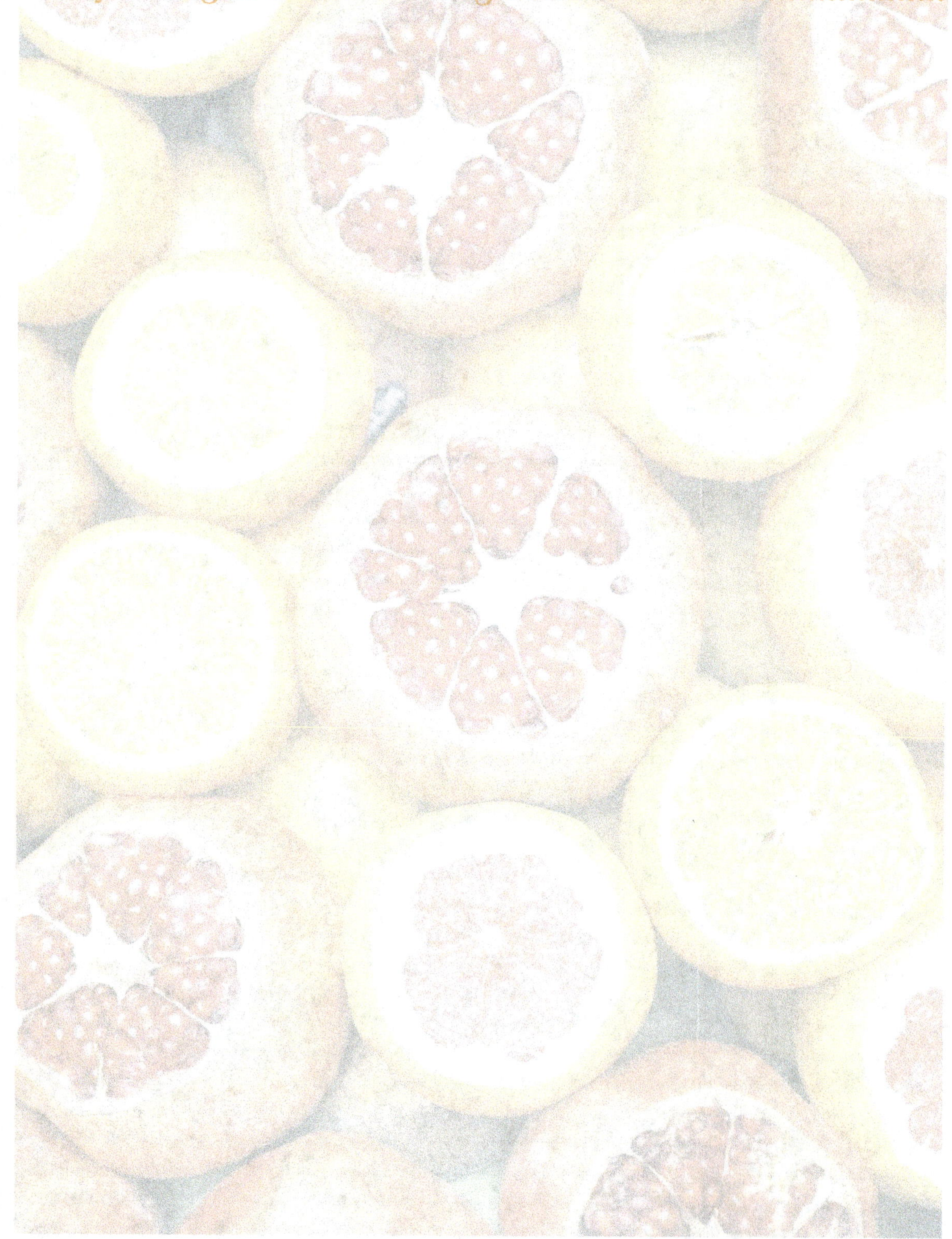

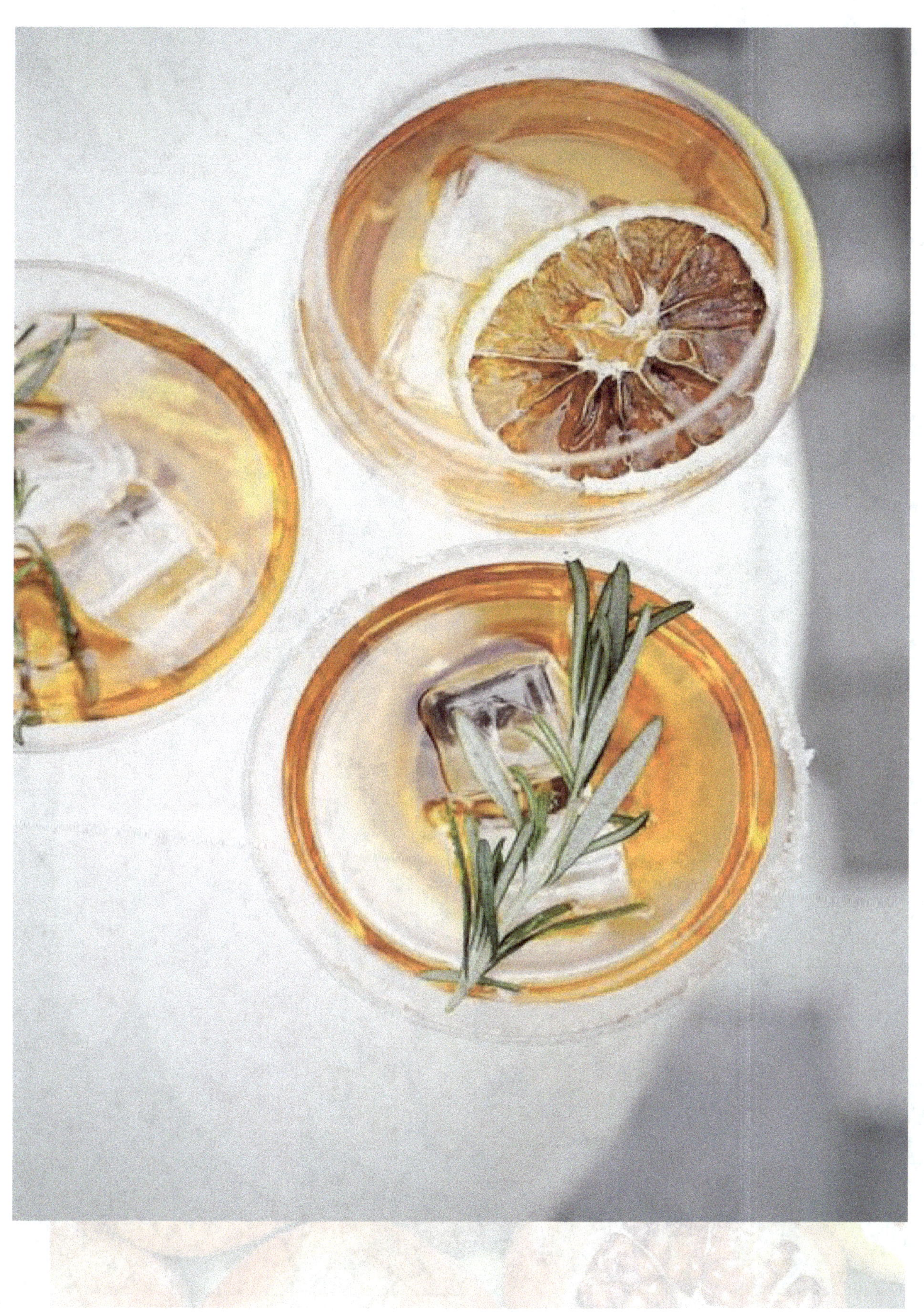

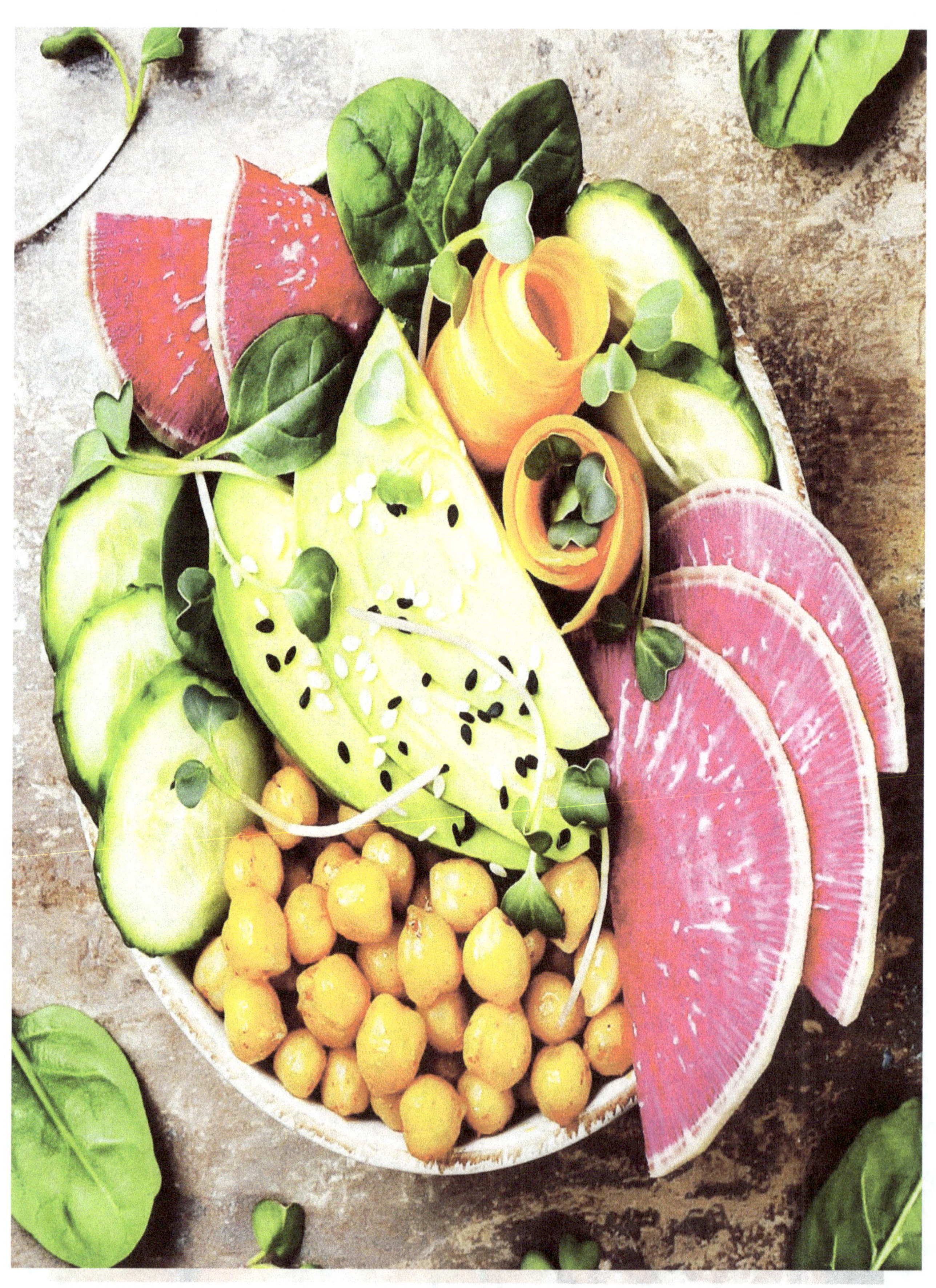

WHAT IS THE PEGAN DIET?

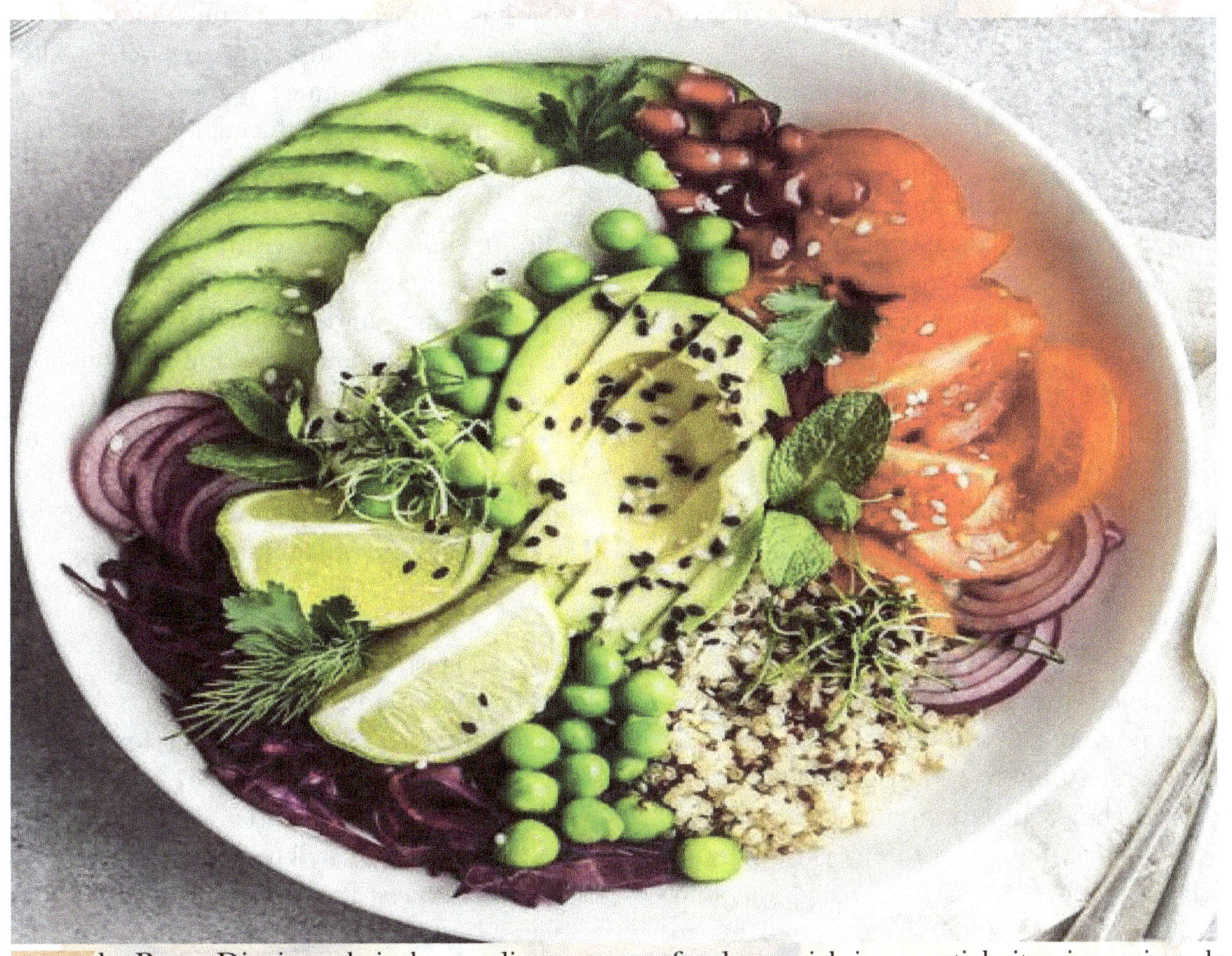

The Pegan Diet is a relatively new dietary concept that combines the best aspects of both the Paleo and Vegan diets. It's a harmonious blend that encourages a balanced approach to eating, focusing on whole, unprocessed foods that promote health and wellness.

At its core, the Pegan Diet emphasizes a plant-based foundation, making vegetables and fruits the star of every meal. This means filling your plate with a colorful array of produce, from leafy greens and vibrant berries to crunchy carrots and juicy tomatoes. These foods are rich in essential vitamins, minerals, and antioxidants that support overall health.

But the Pegan Diet doesn't stop at plants. Unlike a strict vegan diet, it also includes moderate amounts of high-quality animal proteins. This means you can enjoy grass-fed meats, pasture-raised poultry, and wild-caught fish, which provide essential nutrients like omega-3 fatty acids, iron, and B vitamins. The key here is to choose sustainably sourced and ethically raised options.

Healthy fats are another cornerstone of the Pegan Diet. Avocados, nuts, seeds, and olive oil are all encouraged, providing your body with the good fats it needs to thrive. These fats are crucial for brain health, hormone balance, and satiety, helping you feel full and satisfied after meals.

The Pegan Diet also takes a mindful approach to carbohydrates and sugars. While it includes healthy, whole-food sources of carbs like sweet potatoes, quinoa, and legumes, it advises limiting refined grains and sugars. This helps to stabilize blood sugar levels, reduce inflammation, and prevent energy crashes.

One of the most appealing aspects of the Pegan Diet is its flexibility. It doesn't demand strict adherence to a rigid set of rules. Instead, it encourages mindful eating and listening to your body's needs. It's about finding a balance that works for you and making sustainable, healthy choices most of the time.

In essence, the Pegan Diet is about eating clean, nutrient-dense foods that nourish your body and support optimal health. It's a lifestyle choice that promotes longevity and well-being, allowing you to enjoy a variety of delicious foods while staying aligned with your health goals. Whether you're looking to improve your diet, boost your energy, or simply eat more mindfully, the Pegan Diet offers a practical and enjoyable path to better health.

Benefits of a Pegan Lifestyle

Embracing the Pegan lifestyle is more than just following a diet; it's about making mindful choices that prioritize your health and well-being. Here are some of the key benefits of adopting this balanced approach to eating:

1. Nutrient-Dense Diet:

The Pegan diet emphasizes whole, unprocessed foods that are rich in essential nutrients. By focusing on vegetables, fruits, nuts, seeds, and quality proteins, you're ensuring your body receives a diverse array of vitamins, minerals, and antioxidants. This nutrient density supports overall health, boosts your immune system, and helps maintain energy levels throughout the day.

2. Reduced Inflammation:

Chronic inflammation is linked to various health issues, including heart disease, diabetes, and autoimmune disorders. The Pegan diet's emphasis on anti-inflammatory foods, such as leafy greens, fatty fish, nuts, and seeds, can help reduce inflammation in the body. By avoiding processed foods, sugars, and unhealthy fats, you're taking proactive steps to minimize inflammatory responses.

3. Improved Digestion:

A Pegan lifestyle encourages the consumption of fiber-rich foods like vegetables, fruits, and whole grains. Fiber is essential for healthy digestion, as it promotes regular bowel movements and supports a balanced gut microbiome. A well-functioning digestive system is crucial for nutrient absorption and overall health.

4. Balanced Blood Sugar Levels:

One of the cornerstones of the Pegan diet is managing carbohydrate intake and focusing on low-glycemic foods. This approach helps prevent blood sugar spikes and crashes, reducing the risk of type 2 diabetes and promoting steady energy levels. By choosing complex carbs and pairing them with healthy fats and proteins, you can maintain balanced blood sugar levels throughout the day.

5. Heart Health:

The Pegan diet's emphasis on healthy fats from sources like avocados, nuts, seeds, and olive oil supports cardiovascular health. These fats help reduce bad cholesterol levels (LDL) and increase good cholesterol levels (HDL). Additionally, the diet's focus on omega-3 fatty acids from fish and flaxseeds contributes to heart health by reducing inflammation and supporting proper heart function.

6. Sustainable Weight Management:

By prioritizing whole foods and avoiding processed junk, the Pegan diet naturally supports healthy weight management. The diet's balanced approach to macronutrients – including proteins, fats, and carbohydrates – helps you feel satiated and reduces the likelihood of overeating. Over time, this can lead to sustainable weight loss or maintenance without the need for restrictive dieting.

7. Enhanced Mental Clarity:

The nutrient-rich foods promoted in the Pegan lifestyle provide essential vitamins and minerals that support brain health. Omega-3 fatty acids, antioxidants, and other nutrients found in this diet can improve cognitive function, enhance memory, and boost overall mental clarity. By fueling your brain with the right foods, you can experience improved focus and mental sharpness.

8. Ethical and Environmental Considerations:

The Pegan diet encourages a mindful approach to food choices that consider environmental sustainability and animal welfare. By focusing on plant-based foods and choosing responsibly sourced animal products, you can reduce your ecological footprint and support more humane farming practices. This conscious way of eating aligns with values of sustainability and compassion.

9. Flexibility and Personalization:

One of the most appealing aspects of the Pegan lifestyle is its flexibility. Unlike many restrictive diets, the Pegan approach allows for personalization based on individual preferences and needs. Whether you're more inclined towards plant-based eating or prefer a balance with quality animal proteins, the Pegan diet can be adapted to suit your lifestyle.

Adopting the Pegan lifestyle is a holistic approach to health that goes beyond mere nutrition. It's about making thoughtful choices that nurture your body, mind, and spirit, ultimately leading to a more vibrant and balanced life.

HOW TO TRANSITION TO A PEGAN DIET

Transitioning to a Pegan Diet can be an exciting and beneficial journey towards better health and well-being. Here's a human-friendly guide to help you make this transition smoothly

- ❖ **Understanding the Pegan Diet**: Before diving in, it's important to grasp the principles of the Pegan Diet. It combines the best aspects of the Paleo and Vegan diets, focusing on whole, nutrient-dense foods while minimizing processed ingredients.

- ❖ **Start Gradually**: Transitioning doesn't have to be abrupt. Begin by incorporating more plant-based meals into your current diet while reducing processed foods and sugars. This gradual approach allows your taste buds and body to adjust.

- ❖ **Embrace Variety**: One of the strengths of the Pegan Diet is its emphasis on a wide variety of fruits, vegetables, nuts, seeds, and healthy fats. Experiment with different recipes and ingredients to discover what you enjoy the most.

- ❖ **Focus on Quality**: Opt for high-quality, organic produce and sustainably sourced animal products when possible. This ensures you're getting the most nutrients and minimizing exposure to harmful chemicals.

- ❖ **Modify Your Plate**: As you transition, aim to fill your plate with about 75% plant-based foods like leafy greens, colorful vegetables, and fruits. The remaining 25% can include high-quality proteins such as grass-fed meat, wild-caught fish, or organic eggs.

- ❖ **Learn Pegan Cooking** Techniques: Explore new cooking methods that align with the Pegan Diet, such as steaming, sautéing with healthy oils, and using herbs and spices for flavor instead of excessive salt or sugar.

- ❖ **Stay Hydrated**: Water is crucial for overall health and digestion. Make sure to drink plenty of water throughout the day, and consider herbal teas or infused waters for added variety.

- ❖ **Listen to Your Body**: Everyone's nutritional needs are unique. Pay attention to how your body responds to different foods. This awareness can help you tailor your Pegan diet to best suit your individual health goals.

- ❖ **Seek Support**: Transitioning to any new diet can be easier with support from friends, family, or online communities. Share your experiences, recipes, and challenges, and learn from others who are also exploring the Pegan lifestyle.

- ❖ **Be Patient and Flexible**: Rome wasn't built in a day, and neither is a dietary shift. Allow yourself time to adjust and be flexible with your approach. Small changes over time can lead to significant long-term benefits.

- ❖ **Celebrate Successes**: Recognize and celebrate your achievements along the way, whether it's trying a new Pegan recipe, feeling more energetic, or achieving your health goals.

THE FOUNDATIONS OF PEGAN EATING

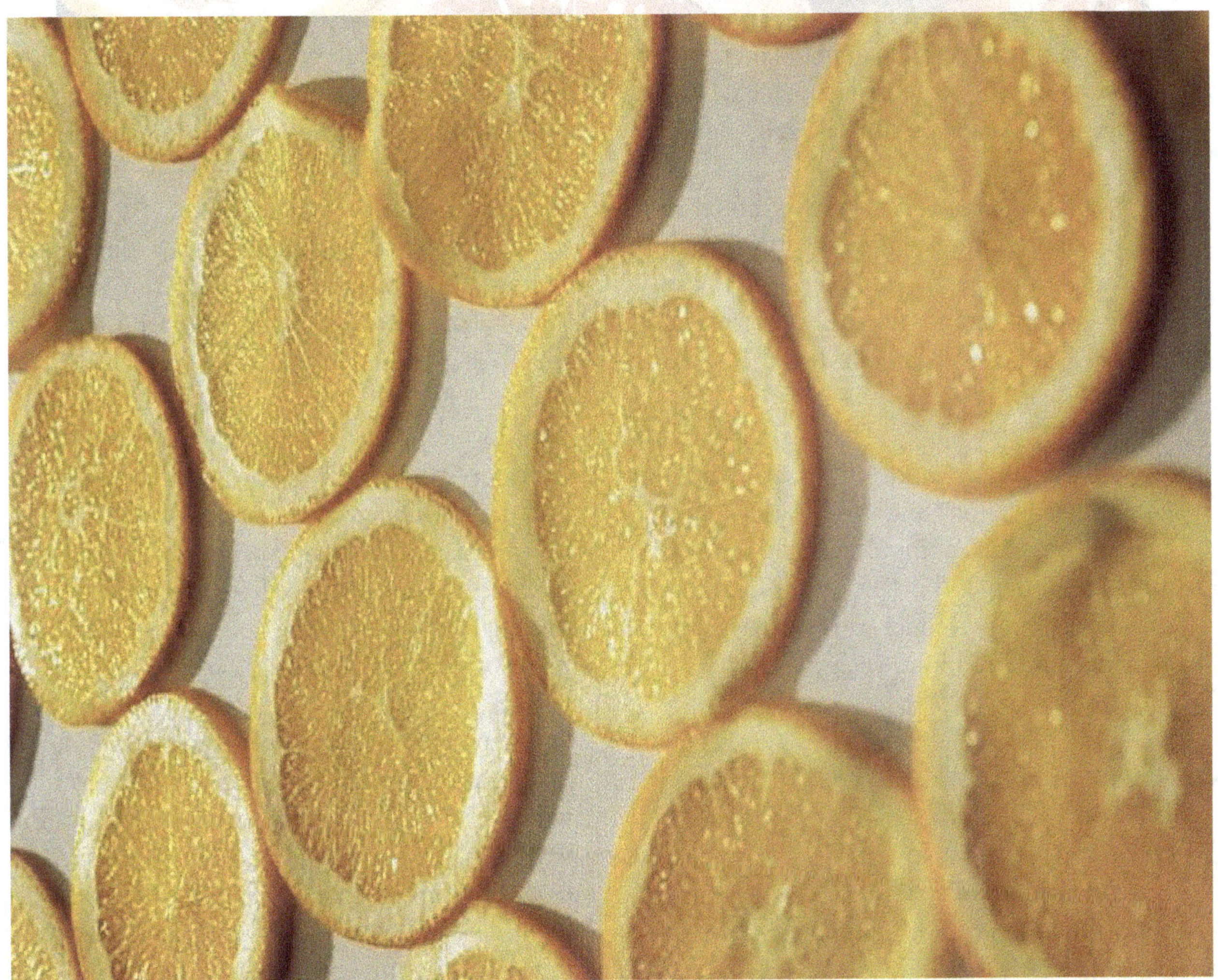

Peganism, at its core, blends the best of two dietary philosophies—Paleo and veganism—creating a balanced approach that prioritizes whole foods and nutrient density. Unlike strict Paleo or vegan diets, Pegan eating encourages flexibility and focuses on what truly nourishes the body.

At the heart of Pegan eating are several foundational principles:

❖ **Emphasis on Whole, Real Foods**: Peganism champions the consumption of whole foods in their natural state. This means opting for fresh vegetables, fruits, nuts, seeds, lean proteins, and healthy fats over processed and refined foods.

❖ **Prioritizing Plant Foods**: Plant-based nutrition forms a significant part of the Pegan diet. It encourages a colorful array of vegetables and fruits, which are rich in vitamins, minerals, antioxidants, and fiber essential for overall health.

❖ **Inclusion of Quality Animal Proteins**: Unlike strict vegan diets, Peganism allows for the inclusion of high-quality animal proteins like grass-fed meats, pasture-raised poultry, and wild-caught fish. These sources provide essential nutrients like omega-3 fatty acids, vitamin B12, and iron.

❖ **Healthy Fats**: Healthy fats are essential in Pegan eating, sourced from foods like avocados, nuts, seeds, and olive oil. These fats support brain function, hormone balance, and overall cellular health.

❖ **Mindful Carbohydrates**: Peganism advocates for mindful carbohydrate consumption, focusing on low-glycemic options such as quinoa, sweet potatoes, and legumes. These carbohydrates provide sustained energy levels without causing spikes in blood sugar.

❖ **Avoidance of Harmful Ingredients**: Pegan eating steers clear of additives, preservatives, and artificial sweeteners commonly found in processed foods. Instead, it encourages reading labels and choosing foods with minimal ingredients.

❖ **Focus on Nutrient Density**: Every meal in the Pegan diet aims to maximize nutrient density, ensuring that each bite contributes significantly to overall health and well-being.

Emphasizing Plant-Based Nutrition

In the world of Peganism, plant-based nutrition takes center stage, offering a wealth of health benefits while promoting environmental sustainability. The core principle of emphasizing plant-based foods revolves around incorporating a diverse array of fruits, vegetables, nuts, seeds, whole grains, and legumes into your daily diet.

Plant-based foods are rich in essential vitamins, minerals, fiber, and antioxidants, which are vital for supporting overall health and well-being. They contribute to lower cholesterol levels, reduced risk of heart disease, and improved digestion. By focusing on plants, Peganism encourages a diet that is naturally low in unhealthy fats and processed sugars, promoting weight management and enhancing energy levels.

Moreover, plants are a sustainable source of nutrition, requiring fewer resources like water and land compared to animal-based foods. This aspect aligns with the Pegan philosophy of mindful eating, where food choices not only benefit personal health but also contribute positively to the planet.

In practical terms, embracing plant-based nutrition means filling your plate with a variety of colorful vegetables and fruits, incorporating whole grains like quinoa and brown rice, and opting for plant-based proteins such as tofu, legumes, and nuts. This approach not only diversifies your nutrient intake but also introduces exciting flavors and textures to your meals.

By making plants the cornerstone of your diet within the Pegan framework, you're not just eating for health but also for a sustainable future—one meal at a time.

Incorporating Quality Animal Proteins

In the Pegan diet, the focus on quality animal proteins emphasizes sourcing from ethical and sustainable practices. This approach not only supports your nutritional needs but also aligns with principles of environmental responsibility and animal welfare.

Choosing quality animal proteins means opting for grass-fed beef, free-range poultry, and wild-caught fish whenever possible. These choices are rich in essential nutrients like omega-3 fatty acids, vitamins, and minerals, contributing to overall health and well-being. By selecting meats and seafood from responsible sources, you can enjoy meals that are not only delicious but also support sustainable agricultural practices and marine conservation efforts.

Balancing these proteins with a predominantly plant-based diet ensures that you receive a diverse array of nutrients while minimizing the environmental impact of your food choices. Whether it's a grilled salmon fillet, a serving of pasture-raised chicken, or occasional lean cuts of beef, integrating these proteins thoughtfully into your meals can enhance both flavor and nutritional value.

Moreover, incorporating quality animal proteins in moderation within a Pegan framework encourages a balanced approach to eating, supporting both personal health goals and sustainable food systems. This mindful approach to protein consumption underscores the Pegan philosophy's commitment to both personal and planetary health, promoting a harmonious relationship with food and the environment.

Balancing Healthy Fats

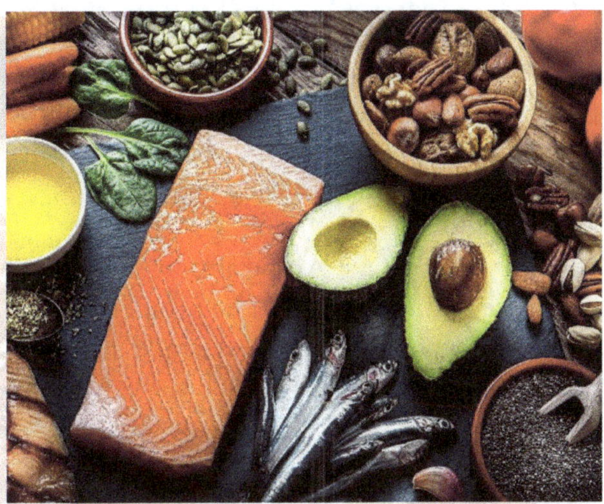

In the world of nutrition, fats often get a bad rap, but not all fats are created equal. Balancing healthy fats is crucial for a well-rounded diet, especially in the Pegan lifestyle. Here's a closer look at how to incorporate healthy fats into your meals in a balanced and nutritious way.

Understanding Healthy Fats;Healthy fats are essential for various bodily functions, including hormone production, brain health, and absorption of fat-soluble vitamins like A, D, E, and K. They also provide a source of long-lasting energy and help keep you feeling satisfied after meals.

Types of Healthy Fats

Monounsaturated fats: Found in foods like avocados, olive oil, and nuts, monounsaturated fats can help reduce bad cholesterol levels and lower the risk of heart disease.

Polyunsaturated fats: Omega-3 and Omega-6 fatty acids fall into this category, which are crucial for brain function and inflammation control. Sources include fatty fish (salmon, mackerel), flaxseeds, chia seeds, and walnuts.

Saturated fats: While traditionally viewed as less healthy, some saturated fats can be part of a balanced diet, particularly those from natural sources like coconut oil and grass-fed dairy products. Moderation is key here.

Avoiding trans fats: Artificial trans fats found in processed foods should be avoided as they increase bad cholesterol levels and raise the risk of heart disease.

Incorporating Healthy Fats into Your Diet

Cooking oils: Choose olive oil, avocado oil, or coconut oil for cooking and salad dressings. These oils are rich in monounsaturated fats and provide a flavorful base for many dishes.

Nuts and seeds: Snack on almonds, walnuts, chia seeds, and flaxseeds for a healthy dose of omega-3 and omega-6 fatty acids. Sprinkle them on salads or yogurt for added crunch and nutrition.

Avocados: Enjoy avocados sliced on toast, blended into smoothies, or as a creamy addition to salads. They are packed with monounsaturated fats, fiber, and essential vitamins.

Fatty fish: Incorporate salmon, sardines, or trout into your meals a few times a week for a rich source of omega-3 fatty acids, which support heart health and brain function.

Managing Carbohydrates and Sugars

In the realm of the Pegan diet, navigating carbohydrates and sugars is crucial for maintaining balance and promoting overall health. Unlike some traditional dietary approaches that demonize all carbs, the Pegan philosophy emphasizes choosing the right kinds of carbohydrates and being mindful of sugar intake.

Choosing the Right Carbohydrates: Carbohydrates are essential for providing energy and supporting bodily functions. However, not all carbs are created equal. The Pegan diet encourages opting for complex carbohydrates found in whole, unprocessed foods like fruits, vegetables, legumes, and whole grains. These foods are rich in fiber, vitamins, and minerals, which contribute to sustained energy levels and overall well-being.

Focusing on Fiber: Fiber plays a pivotal role in the Pegan diet by slowing down the absorption of sugars into the bloodstream and promoting digestive health. Foods such as leafy greens, broccoli, berries, and nuts are excellent sources of fiber. Including these in your daily meals helps in managing blood sugar levels and supporting weight management goals.

Limiting Added Sugars: While natural sugars found in fruits are welcomed in moderation on the Pegan diet, added sugars found in processed foods and beverages should be limited. These sugars can lead to spikes in blood sugar levels and contribute to health issues like obesity and diabetes. Opting for natural sweeteners like honey or maple syrup sparingly, or better yet, enjoying the natural sweetness of whole fruits, aligns with Pegan principles.

Balancing Carbohydrates with Proteins and Fats: In Pegan meals, balance is key. Combining carbohydrates with healthy fats and lean proteins helps in slowing down digestion, keeping you fuller for longer, and stabilizing energy levels throughout the day. For example, pairing quinoa (a complex carbohydrate) with grilled chicken and a side of leafy greens provides a well-rounded meal that supports both physical and mental clarity.

Practical Tips for Managing Carbohydrates and Sugars:

Read Labels: Be mindful of hidden sugars and processed ingredients in packaged foods.

Cook at Home: Prepare meals from scratch using whole ingredients to control sugar content.

Moderation is Key: Enjoy treats occasionally while focusing primarily on nutrient-dense foods.

Stay Hydrated: Drinking plenty of water supports healthy digestion and metabolism.

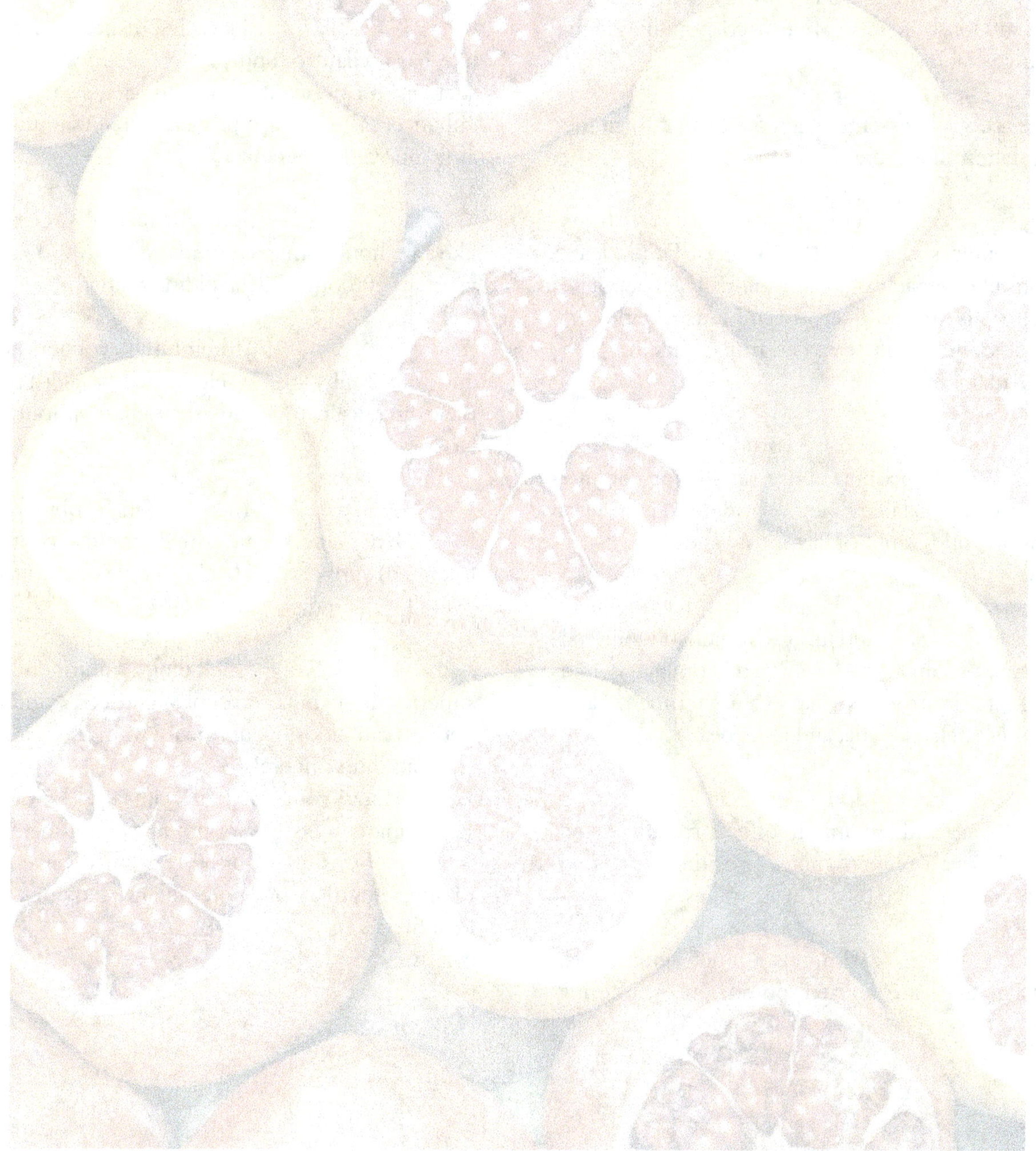

ESSENTIAL PEGAN INGREDIENTS

Embarking on a Pegan diet means stocking your pantry with wholesome ingredients that nourish both body and soul. The Pegan approach blends the best of two dietary worlds: emphasizing nutrient-dense plants while incorporating high-quality proteins.

Here are some essential ingredients that form the foundation of a Pegan kitchen:

1. Fresh Produce: Vibrant vegetables and fruits take center stage in a Pegan diet. Think leafy greens like spinach and kale, colorful bell peppers, cruciferous veggies like broccoli and cauliflower, and a rainbow of seasonal fruits bursting with antioxidants.

2. Healthy Oils and Fats: Avocado oil, extra virgin olive oil, and coconut oil are staples for cooking and dressing salads. They provide essential fatty acids and add depth of flavor to dishes.

3. Quality Proteins: Pegan meals include lean meats like chicken and turkey, sustainably sourced fish such as salmon and trout rich in omega-3s, and plant-based proteins like tofu, tempeh, and legumes such as lentils and chickpeas.

4. Whole Grains and Pseudocereals: Quinoa, buckwheat, and amaranth offer protein-packed alternatives to refined grains, providing sustained energy without the blood sugar spikes.

5. Nuts and Seeds: Almonds, walnuts, chia seeds, and flaxseeds are nutrient powerhouses, offering protein, healthy fats, and fiber. They're perfect for adding crunch to salads or blending into smoothies.

6. Herbs and Spices: Flavoring dishes with herbs like basil, cilantro, and parsley, along with spices such as turmeric, cumin, and ginger, not only enhances taste but also provides anti-inflammatory and antioxidant benefits.

7. Natural Sweeteners: Opt for natural sweeteners like raw honey, maple syrup, and dates to satisfy your sweet tooth while avoiding refined sugars.

8. Non-Dairy Milks: Almond milk, coconut milk, and oat milk are excellent dairy alternatives, providing calcium and vitamins without the lactose.

9. Fermented Foods: Incorporating probiotic-rich foods like sauerkraut, kimchi, and yogurt (if tolerated) supports gut health, aiding digestion and overall well-being.

10. Superfoods: Including nutrient-dense superfoods such as spirulina, chia seeds, and acai berries can boost your meals with antioxidants, vitamins, and minerals.

By stocking your kitchen with these essential Pegan ingredients, you're not just preparing meals – you're nourishing your body with a diverse array of nutrients that promote vitality and long-term health.

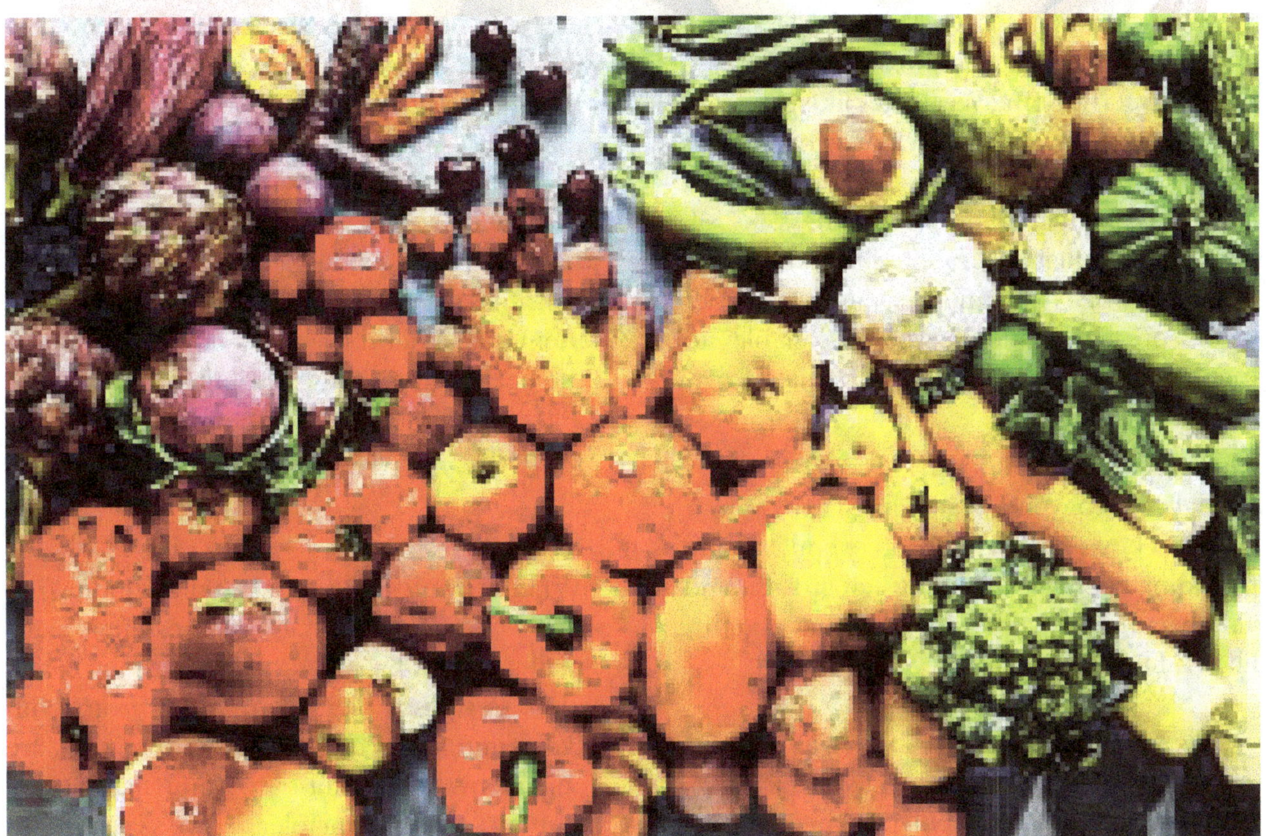

In the world of Pegan eating, fresh produce takes center stage as a cornerstone of nutritious and vibrant meals. Vegetables and fruits not only add color and flavor to dishes but also provide essential vitamins, minerals, fiber, and antioxidants that support overall health and well-being.

Why Fresh Produce Matters: Including a variety of vegetables and fruits in your diet ensures you get a diverse range of nutrients. From leafy greens like spinach and kale packed with iron and vitamins A, C, and K, to colorful bell peppers rich in antioxidants, each vegetable offers unique health benefits. Fruits such as berries, citrus fruits, and apples provide natural sweetness along with vitamins, fiber, and phytonutrients that help boost immunity and promote digestion.

Choosing the Best: Opt for locally grown, seasonal produce when possible, as they tend to be fresher and more flavorful. Whether shopping at farmers' markets or grocery stores, look for vibrant colors and firm textures, indicating freshness. Experiment with different varieties to discover new flavors and textures that complement your Pegan meals.

Incorporating into Your Meals: Vegetables and fruits can be enjoyed in various ways in Pegan cooking. They can be roasted, steamed, grilled, or enjoyed raw in salads and wraps. Smoothies and juices are excellent ways to pack in a variety of fruits and leafy greens for a refreshing and nutrient-dense boost. When preparing meals, aim to fill half of your plate with colorful vegetables and fruits to ensure a balanced and satisfying meal.

Storing and Preparing: To maximize freshness and nutritional content, store vegetables and fruits properly. Some vegetables like tomatoes and avocados ripen after picking, while others like leafy greens and berries should be consumed sooner for peak freshness. Wash produce thoroughly before use to remove any pesticides or contaminants, and consider using organic options when available to minimize exposure to harmful chemicals.

Healthy Oils and Fats

In the realm of nutrition, oils and fats play crucial roles beyond just adding flavor to our meals. They are essential for overall health, providing energy, supporting cell growth, and aiding in the absorption of fat-soluble vitamins like A, D, E, and K.

Understanding Healthy Fats: Not all fats are created equal. Healthy fats, such as monounsaturated and polyunsaturated fats, are beneficial for heart health when consumed in moderation. These fats are typically found in foods like avocados, nuts, seeds, and oily fish such as salmon and mackerel. They help lower harmful LDL cholesterol levels and raise beneficial HDL cholesterol levels, reducing the risk of heart disease.

The Role of Omega-3 Fatty Acids: Omega-3 fatty acids, a type of polyunsaturated fat, are particularly renowned for their anti-inflammatory properties and benefits for brain health. Sources of omega-3s include fatty fish (like salmon, sardines, and trout), flaxseeds, chia seeds, and walnuts. Including these in your diet can help support cognitive function and contribute to overall well-being.

Choosing the Right Cooking Oils:

When it comes to cooking, opting for oils with high smoke points, like olive oil, avocado oil, and coconut oil, is important. These oils are more stable at higher temperatures, making them suitable for sautéing, roasting, and even light frying without breaking down and forming harmful compounds.

Balancing Fat Intake: While incorporating healthy fats is beneficial, it's essential to consume them in moderation and balance them with other nutrients. Too much fat, even the healthy kind, can contribute to weight gain and other health issues if not managed properly.

Pegan-Friendly Proteins

When it comes to the Pegan diet, finding the right protein sources is essential for maintaining a balanced and nourishing eating plan. Peganism blends principles from both Paleo and vegan diets, so protein choices are guided by both plant-based and high-quality animal protein principles. Here's a guide to integrating Pegan-friendly proteins into your meals, ensuring you get the nutrients you need without compromising on taste or health.

1. Plant-Based Proteins

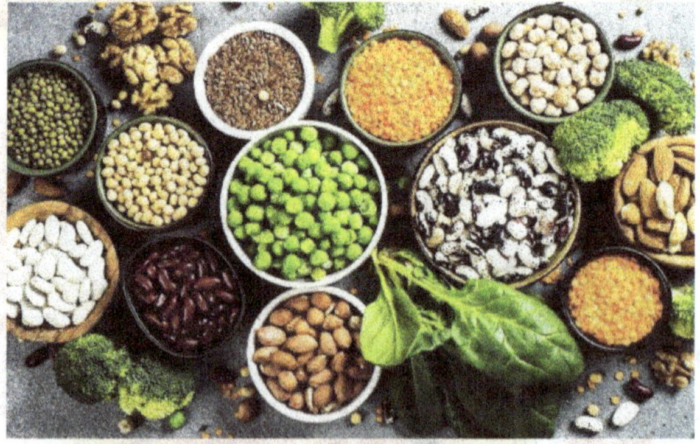

Legumes: Beans, lentils, and chickpeas are fantastic sources of plant-based protein. They are versatile and can be used in a variety of dishes—from hearty soups to vibrant salads. These legumes not only provide protein but also offer fiber, which is crucial for digestive health.

Nuts and Seeds: Almonds, walnuts, chia seeds, flaxseeds, and hemp seeds are nutrient-dense and protein-rich. They make great snacks, toppings for salads, or can be blended into smoothies. Their healthy fats also support heart health and provide a good source of energy.

Quinoa: Often considered a complete protein because it contains all nine essential amino acids, quinoa is a great addition to any Pegan meal. Use it as a base for salads, a side dish, or even breakfast porridge.

Edamame: These young soybeans are not only a protein powerhouse but also packed with vitamins and minerals. They can be enjoyed as a snack, added to salads, or included in stir-fries.

2. High-Quality Animal Proteins

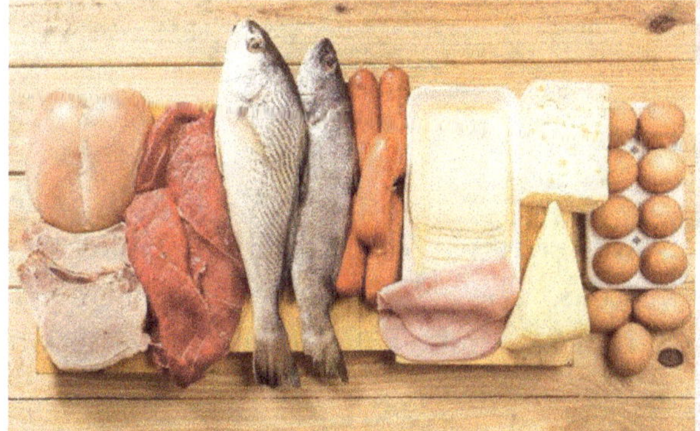

Grass-Fed Meats: Beef from grass-fed cows is a great source of protein and tends to have a better nutritional profile compared to grain-fed options. It's richer in omega-3 fatty acids and antioxidants. Opt for lean cuts and use them in moderation as part of a balanced diet.

Free-Range Poultry: Chicken and turkey that are pasture-raised or free-range offer high-quality protein while avoiding antibiotics and hormones. They're versatile for various recipes, from roasted dishes to salads.

Wild-Caught Fish: Fish such as salmon, mackerel, and sardines are rich in protein and provide essential omega-3 fatty acids. Wild-caught varieties are preferred over farmed for their better nutritional profile and lower environmental impact.

Eggs: For those who include animal products, eggs are an excellent source of complete protein and nutrients. Opt for eggs from free-range or pasture-raised chickens for a healthier option.

3. Balancing Proteins

Incorporating Pegan-friendly proteins involves balancing plant-based options with high-quality animal proteins. This not only ensures you meet your protein needs but also provides a variety of nutrients essential for overall health. Remember, moderation and variety are key. Combining different sources of protein throughout your meals will help you enjoy a rich and satisfying Pegan diet while reaping the benefits of diverse nutritional sources.

Avoiding Processed and Refined Foods

In today's fast-paced world, it's easy to reach for convenience foods that promise a quick meal or snack. However, these processed and refined foods often come at a hidden cost to our health. Embracing a Pegan lifestyle means making conscious choices to nourish our bodies with whole, natural foods, steering clear of those that have been altered or stripped of their nutritional value.

Processed foods are typically altered from their natural state through various methods such as adding preservatives, flavorings, and other additives. These modifications often enhance flavor, extend shelf life, and make food more convenient to prepare. However, this convenience can be deceptive. Many processed foods are high in unhealthy fats, sugars, and sodium, contributing to a host of health problems like obesity, heart disease, and diabetes.

Refined foods, on the other hand, have been stripped of their original, natural elements. For example, white flour is made by removing the bran and germ from the wheat, leaving behind a product with significantly less fiber, vitamins, and minerals. Similarly, refined sugar is extracted and purified, losing the beneficial nutrients found in natural sources like fruits and vegetables.

So why should we avoid these foods? Here are a few compelling reasons:

Nutritional Deficiency: Processed and refined foods are often low in essential nutrients. They might provide calories, but they lack the vitamins, minerals, and fiber that whole foods offer. Over time, relying on these foods can lead to deficiencies that impact overall health.

Empty Calories: Many processed foods are calorie-dense but nutrient-poor. This means they can contribute to weight gain without providing the necessary nutrients to keep our bodies functioning optimally. It's a classic case of eating a lot but still feeling unsatisfied and hungry.

Additives and Preservatives: Processed foods often contain artificial additives and preservatives, which can have negative effects on health. Some people may experience allergic reactions or other adverse effects from these substances. Additionally, the long-term impact of consuming large amounts of these additives is still not fully understood.

Blood Sugar Spikes: Refined foods, especially those high in sugar, can cause rapid spikes and crashes in blood sugar levels. This can lead to cravings, mood swings, and energy slumps, making it harder to maintain a balanced diet and healthy weight.

Increased Risk of Chronic Diseases: Diets high in processed and refined foods have been linked to an increased risk of chronic diseases such as heart disease, diabetes, and cancer. By reducing or eliminating these foods from our diet, we can lower our risk and promote better long-term health.

Embracing a Pegan lifestyle involves choosing whole, unprocessed foods whenever possible. Here are some tips to help you make the transition:

- Focus on Fresh Produce: Fill your plate with a variety of colorful vegetables and fruits. These foods are rich in vitamins, minerals, and antioxidants that support overall health.

- Choose Whole Grains: Opt for whole grains like quinoa, brown rice, and oats instead of refined grains. Whole grains retain their natural fiber and nutrients, making them a healthier choice.

- Healthy Fats: Incorporate sources of healthy fats such as avocados, nuts, seeds, and olive oil. These fats are essential for brain health and can help keep you feeling full and satisfied.

❖ **Lean Proteins:** Select high-quality, lean proteins like grass-fed meat, free-range poultry, and plant-based options such as beans and lentils. Avoid processed meats, which are often high in unhealthy fats and preservatives.

❖ **Read Labels:** When buying packaged foods, take the time to read ingredient labels. Look for products with minimal, recognizable ingredients and avoid those with long lists of additives and preservatives.

❖ **Cook at Home:** Preparing meals at home gives you control over what goes into your food. Experiment with new recipes and cooking methods to make healthy eating enjoyable and sustainable.

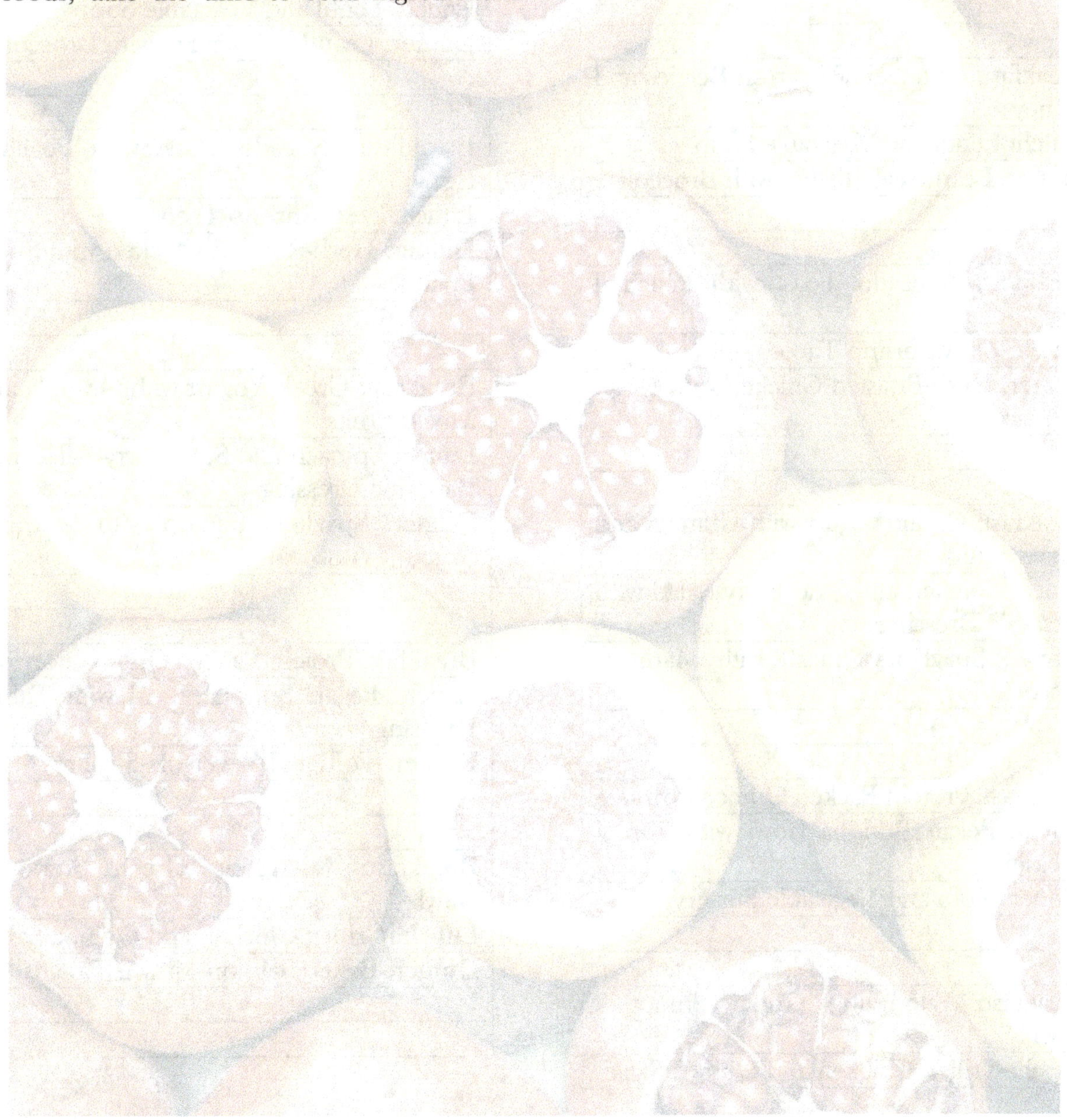

14 DAYS PEGAN MEALS

Day 1:

Breakfast: Energizing Green Smoothie Bowl

Lunch: Grilled Chicken and Quinoa Salad

Dinner: Baked Salmon with Asparagus

Day 2:

Breakfast: Oatmeal with Fresh Berries and Honey

Lunch: Lentil and Vegetable Soup

Dinner: Lean Beef Stir-Fry with Broccoli

Day 3:

Breakfast: Avocado Toast with Poached Egg

Lunch: Zesty Shrimp Tacos

Dinner: Herb-Roasted Chicken with Sweet Potatoes

Day 4:

Breakfast: Greek Yogurt with Granola and Mixed Fruits

Lunch: Spinach and Strawberry Salad with Balsamic Dressing

Dinner: Spaghetti Squash with Marinara Sauce

Day 5:

Breakfast: Protein-Packed Quinoa Porridge

Lunch: Pegan Buddha Bowl with Tahini Dressing

Dinner: Tofu and Vegetable Stir-Fry

Day 6:

Breakfast: Energizing Green Smoothie Bowl

Lunch: Grilled Chicken and Quinoa Salad

Dinner: Baked Salmon with Asparagus

Day 7:

Breakfast: Oatmeal with Fresh Berries and Honey

Lunch: Lentil and Vegetable Soup

Dinner: Lean Beef Stir-Fry with Broccoli

Day 8:

Breakfast: Avocado Toast with Poached Egg

Lunch: Zesty Shrimp Tacos

Dinner: Herb-Roasted Chicken with Sweet Potatoes

Day 9:

Breakfast: Greek Yogurt with Granola and Mixed Fruits

Lunch: Spinach and Strawberry Salad with Balsamic Dressing

Dinner: Spaghetti Squash with Marinara Sauce

Day 10:

Breakfast: Protein-Packed Quinoa Porridge

Lunch: Pegan Buddha Bowl with Tahini Dressing

Dinner: Tofu and Vegetable Stir-Fry

Day 11:

Breakfast: Energizing Green Smoothie Bowl

Lunch: Grilled Chicken and Quinoa Salad

Dinner: Baked Salmon with Asparagus

Day 12:

| Breakfast: Oatmeal with Fresh Berries and Honey |
| Lunch: Lentil and Vegetable Soup |
| Dinner: Lean Beef Stir-Fry with Broccoli |

| Breakfast: Avocado Toast with Poached Egg |
| Lunch: Zesty Shrimp Tacos |
| Dinner: Herb-Roasted Chicken with Sweet Potatoes |

| Breakfast: Greek Yogurt with Granola and Mixed Fruits |
| Lunch: Spinach and Strawberry Salad with Balsamic Dressing |
| Dinner: Spaghetti Squash with Marinara Sauce |

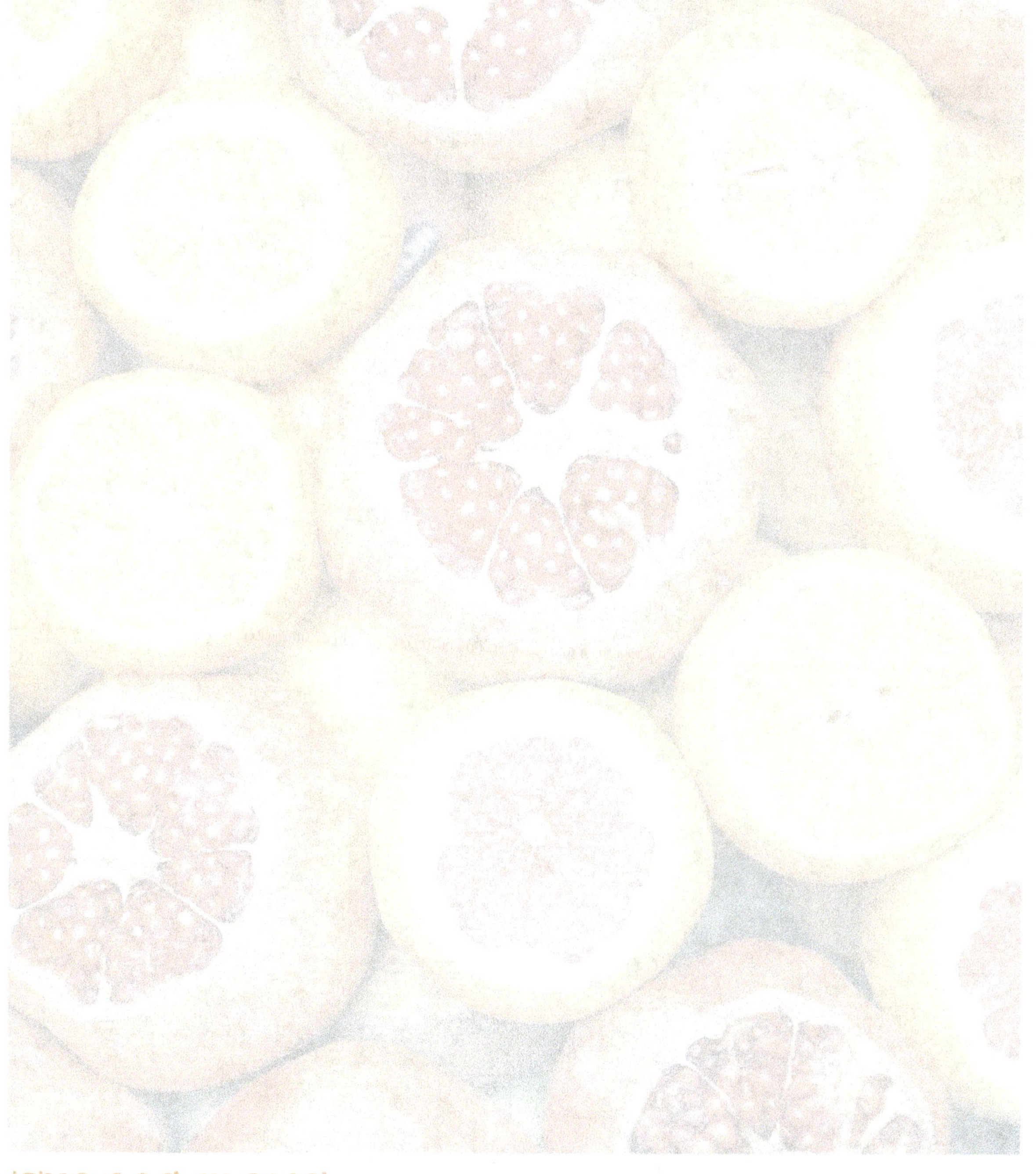

CHAPTER 4: PEGAN BREAKFAST RECIPES

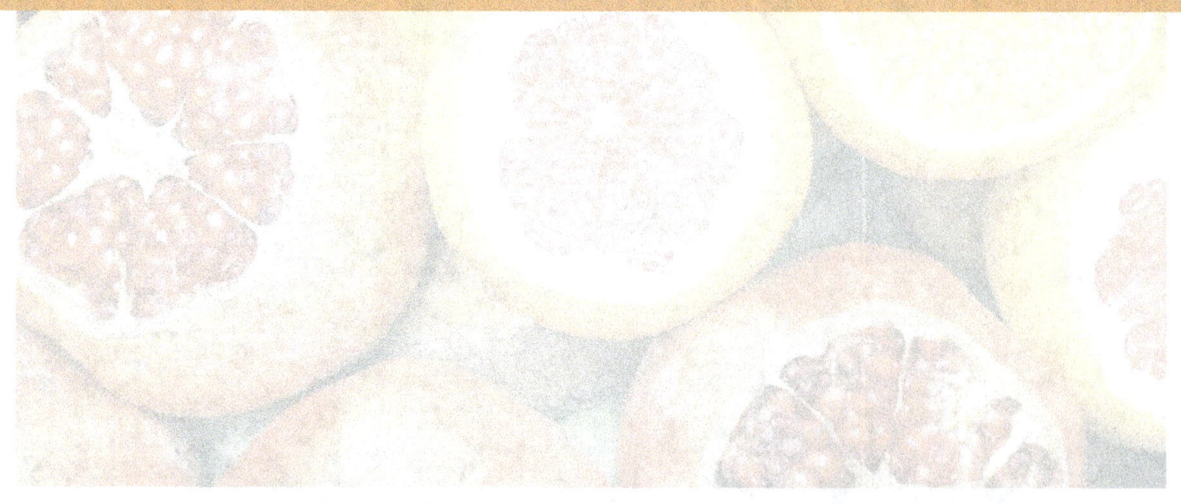

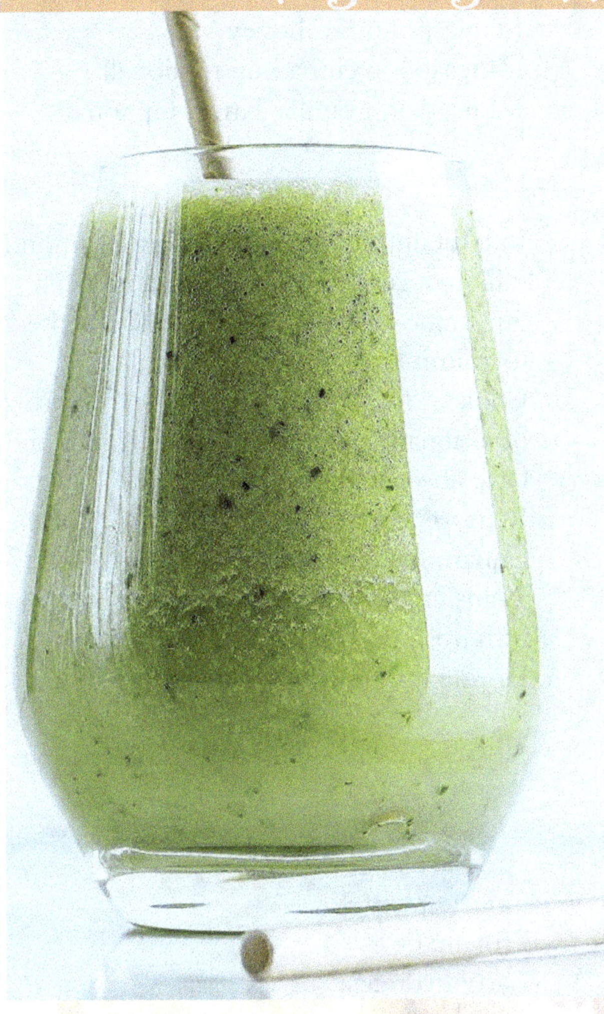

- 1 frozen banana
- 1 cup fresh spinach
- 1/2 avocado
- 1 tablespoon chia seeds
- 1 tablespoon almond butter
- 1/2 cup ice
- Toppings: fresh berries, sliced almonds, coconut flakes, and a drizzle of honey (optional)

Procedure:

- In a blender, combine the almond milk, frozen banana, spinach, avocado, chia seeds, almond butter, and ice.
- Blend until smooth and creamy, adjusting the consistency with more almond milk if necessary.
- Pour the smoothie into a bowl.
- Top with fresh berries, sliced almonds, coconut flakes, and a drizzle of honey, if desired.

Nutritional Information (per serving):

- Calories: 300
- Protein: 7g
- Fat: 18g
- Carbohydrates: 30g
- Fiber: 10g
- Sugars: 10

Preparation Time: 10 minutes

Ingredients:

- 1 cup unsweetened almond milk

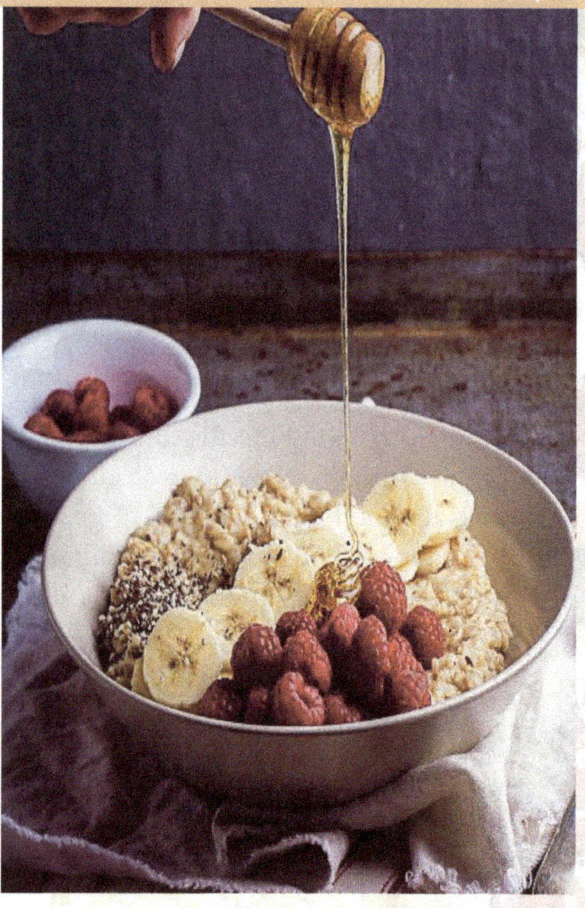

- 1 tablespoon raw honey
- 1/4 teaspoon cinnamon (optional)
- 1/4 teaspoon vanilla extract (optional)

Procedure:

- In a medium saucepan, bring the almond milk to a gentle boil over medium heat.
- Stir in the rolled oats and reduce the heat to a simmer.
- Cook for 5-7 minutes, stirring occasionally, until the oats are tender and have absorbed most of the milk.
- Remove from heat and stir in the cinnamon and vanilla extract, if using.
- Transfer the oatmeal to a bowl and top with fresh berries.
- Drizzle with raw honey before serving.

Nutritional Information (per serving):

- Calories: 250
- Protein: 6g
- Carbohydrates: 45g
- Dietary Fiber: 8g
- Sugars: 15g
- Fat: 4g
- Saturated Fat: 0.5g

Preparation Time: 10 minutes

Ingredients:

- 1 cup rolled oats
- 2 cups almond milk or any non-dairy milk
- 1/2 cup mixed fresh berries (blueberries, strawberries, raspberries)

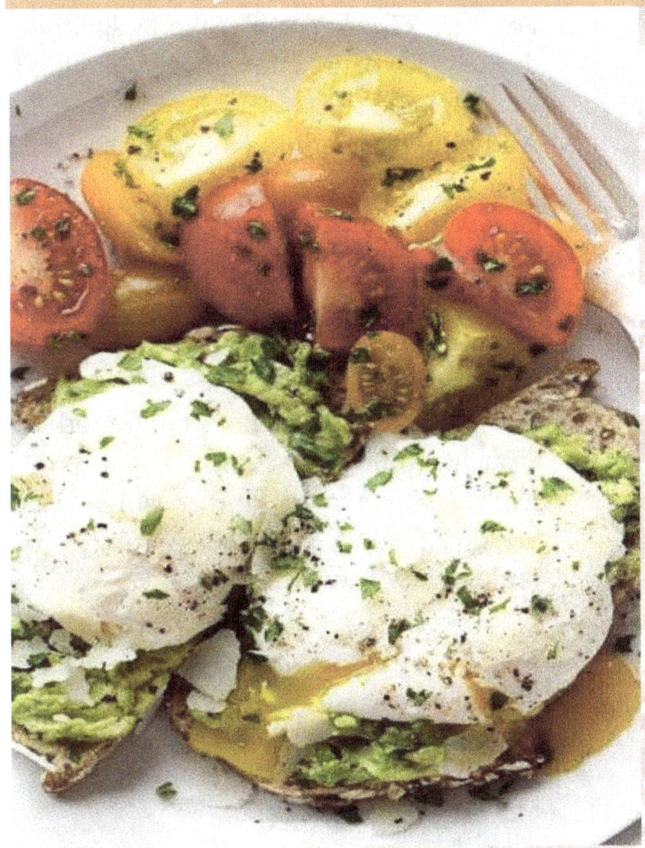

Preparation Time: 15 minutes

Ingredients:

- 1 ripe avocado
- 2 large eggs
- 2 slices of whole-grain or gluten-free bread
- 1 tablespoon lemon juice
- Salt and pepper to taste
- Optional: red pepper flakes, microgreens, or cherry tomatoes for garnish

Procedure:

- Prepare the Avocado: Cut the avocado in half, remove the pit, and scoop the flesh into a bowl. Mash the avocado with a fork until smooth. Add lemon juice, salt, and pepper, and mix well.
- Poach the Eggs: Fill a saucepan with water and bring it to a gentle simmer. Crack each egg into a small bowl. Create a gentle whirlpool in the water with a spoon and carefully slide one egg into the center. Poach for about 3-4 minutes or until the whites are set but the yolk is still runny. Remove with a slotted spoon and repeat with the second egg.
- Toast the Bread: While the eggs are poaching, toast the bread slices to your desired level of crispiness.
- Assemble the Toast: Spread the mashed avocado evenly on each slice of toast. Place a poached egg on top of each slice. Add optional garnishes if desired.
- Season and Serve: Sprinkle with additional salt, pepper, and optional red pepper flakes. Serve immediately.

Nutritional Information (per serving):

- Calories: 350
- Protein: 14g
- Carbohydrates: 30g
- Fat: 20g
- Fiber: 10g

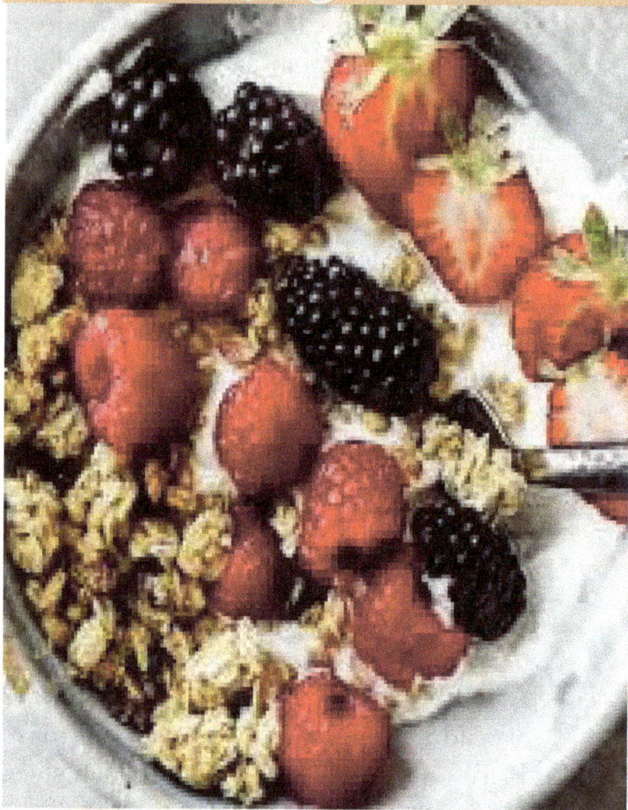

Preparation Time: 5 minutes

Ingredients:

- 1 cup Greek yogurt (dairy-free, if strictly following Pegan principles)
- 1/4 cup granola (grain-free, homemade or store-bought)
- 1/2 cup mixed fresh fruits (e.g., berries, apple slices, banana)
- 1 tablespoon nuts or seeds (optional for extra crunch)
- 1 teaspoon honey or maple syrup (optional for sweetness)

Procedure:

- Layer the Greek Yogurt: Start by spooning the Greek yogurt into a bowl, creating a smooth base.
- Add Granola: Sprinkle the granola evenly over the yogurt.
- Top with Fruits: Arrange the mixed fruits on top of the granola. Use a variety of colors and textures for a visually appealing and nutritious mix.
- Optional Add-Ons: If desired, sprinkle nuts or seeds over the fruit for added crunch and nutrients.
- Drizzle Sweetener: Finish with a light drizzle of honey or maple syrup, if you prefer a bit of sweetness.

Nutritional Information (Approximate):

- Calories: 300
- Protein: 15g
- Fat: 10g
- Carbohydrates: 40g
- Fiber: 5g
- Sugars: 20g

Notes:

- Ensure the granola is grain-free to align with Pegan guidelines.
- Opt for unsweetened Greek yogurt or dairy-free alternatives to keep the dish Pegan-friendly.
- Choose organic, seasonal fruits for the best nutritional value and flavor.

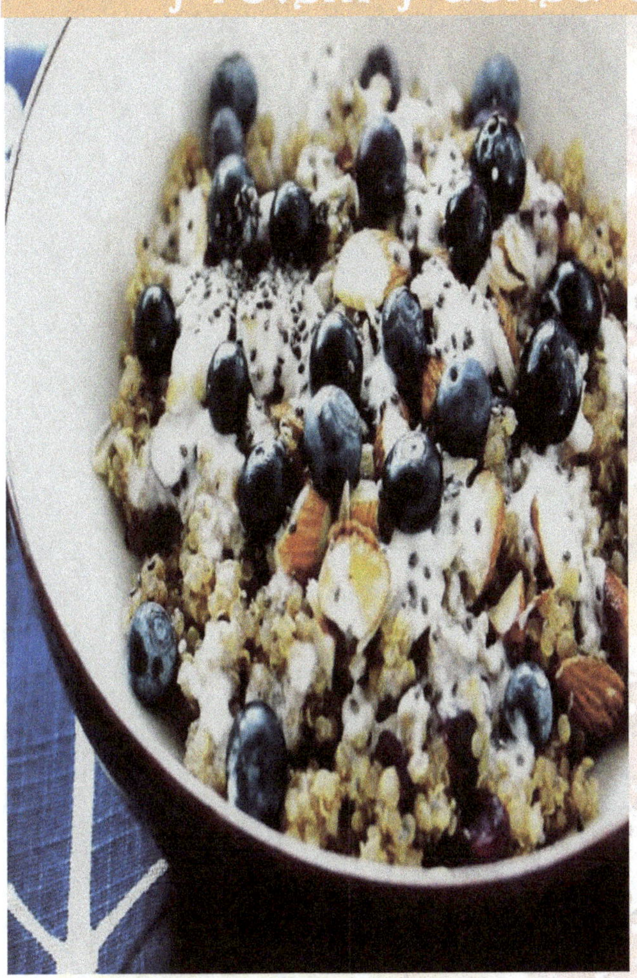

- 1 tablespoon maple syrup (optional)
- Fresh berries, for topping
- Nuts and seeds, for topping

Procedure:

- In a medium saucepan, combine quinoa and almond milk. Bring to a boil over medium heat.
- Reduce heat to low, cover, and simmer for about 15 minutes, or until the quinoa is tender and most of the liquid is absorbed.
- Stir in chia seeds, vanilla extract, and maple syrup (if using). Cook for another 2-3 minutes, until the porridge thickens.
- Remove from heat and let sit for a few minutes to allow the chia seeds to absorb more liquid.
- Serve warm, topped with fresh berries, nuts, and seeds for added texture and flavor.

Nutritional Information (per serving):

- Calories: 250
- Protein: 8g
- Carbohydrates: 40g
- Fiber: 6g
- Sugars: 5g (without maple syrup)
- Fat: 6g

Preparation Time: 20 minutes

Ingredients:

- 1 cup quinoa, rinsed
- 2 cups unsweetened almond milk
- 1 tablespoon chia seeds
- 1 teaspoon vanilla extract

CHAPTER 5:

PEGAN

LUNCH

RECIPES

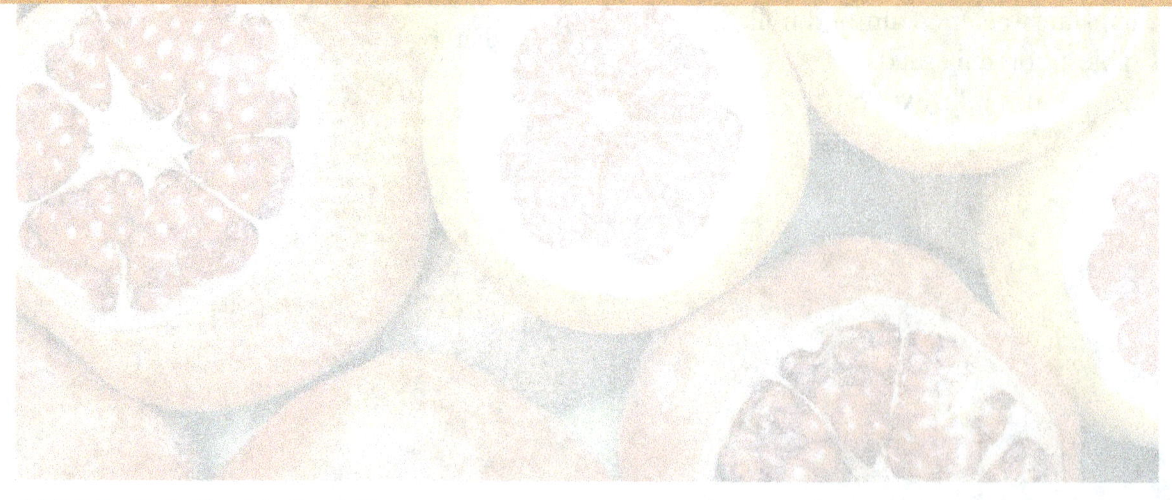

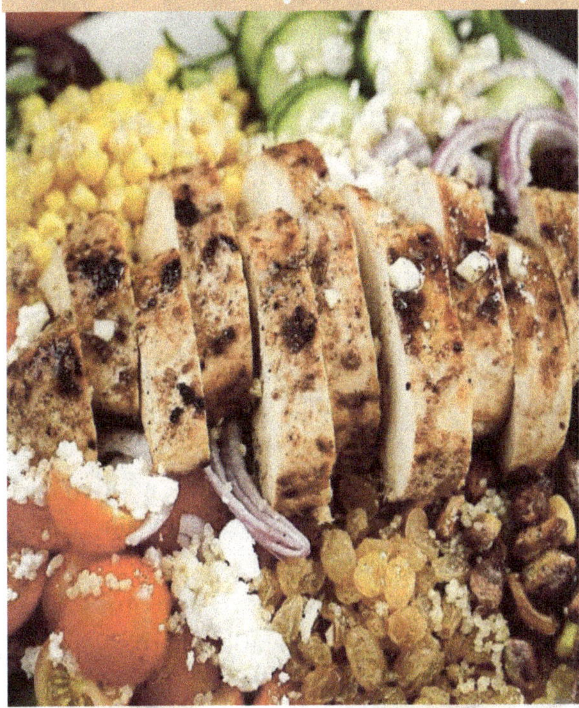

Preparation Time: 30 minutes

Ingredients:

- 1 cup quinoa, rinsed
- 2 cups water
- 2 boneless, skinless chicken breasts
- 1 tablespoon olive oil
- Salt and pepper to taste
- 1 cup cherry tomatoes, halved
- 1 cucumber, diced
- 1 red bell pepper, diced
- 1 avocado, diced
- 2 cups mixed greens
- 1/4 cup fresh parsley, chopped
- Juice of 1 lemon
- 2 tablespoons olive oil (for dressing)
- Salt and pepper (for dressing)

Procedure:

- Cook Quinoa: In a medium saucepan, bring quinoa and water to a boil. Reduce heat, cover, and simmer for 15 minutes or until water is absorbed. Fluff with a fork and set aside.
- Prepare Chicken: While quinoa cooks, preheat grill to medium-high heat. Brush chicken breasts with olive oil and season with salt and pepper. Grill chicken for 6-7 minutes on each side or until fully cooked. Remove from grill and let rest for 5 minutes before slicing.
- Assemble Salad: In a large bowl, combine cooked quinoa, cherry tomatoes, cucumber, bell pepper, avocado, and mixed greens.
- Dress Salad: In a small bowl, whisk together lemon juice, olive oil, salt, and pepper. Pour dressing over salad and toss to combine.
- Serve: Top the salad with sliced grilled chicken and sprinkle with fresh parsley. Serve immediately.

Nutritional Information (per serving):

- Calories: 450
- Protein: 30g
- Carbohydrates: 35g
- Fat: 20g
- Fiber: 8g

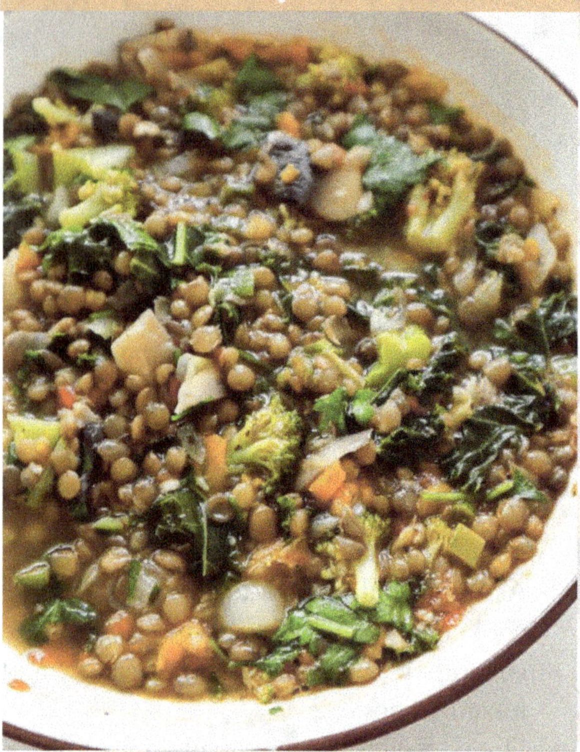

Preparation Time: 45 minutes

Ingredients:

* 1 cup green or brown lentils, rinsed
* 2 tablespoons olive oil
* 1 large onion, chopped
* 2 cloves garlic, minced
* 2 carrots, diced
* 2 celery stalks, diced
* 1 zucchini, diced
* 1 bell pepper, diced
* 1 can (14.5 oz) diced tomatoes
* 6 cups vegetable broth
* 1 teaspoon ground cumin
* 1 teaspoon ground coriander
* 1 teaspoon smoked paprika
* 1 bay leaf
* Salt and pepper to taste
* Fresh spinach or kale, chopped (optional, for added greens)
* Fresh parsley, chopped (for garnish)

Procedure:

* Heat the olive oil in a large pot over medium heat. Add the chopped onion and garlic, and sauté until the onion is translucent, about 5 minutes.
* Add the diced carrots, celery, zucchini, and bell pepper. Cook for another 5-7 minutes, stirring occasionally, until the vegetables start to soften.
* Stir in the lentils, diced tomatoes (with their juice), and vegetable broth.
* Add the ground cumin, ground coriander, smoked paprika, and bay leaf. Season with salt and pepper to taste.
* Bring the soup to a boil, then reduce the heat and let it simmer for 25-30 minutes, or until the lentils are tender.
* If using, stir in the chopped spinach or kale during the last 5 minutes of cooking.
* Remove the bay leaf before serving. Garnish with fresh parsley.

Nutritional Information (per serving):

* Calories: 220
* Protein: 12g
* Carbohydrates: 35g
* Fiber: 12g
* Fat: 5g

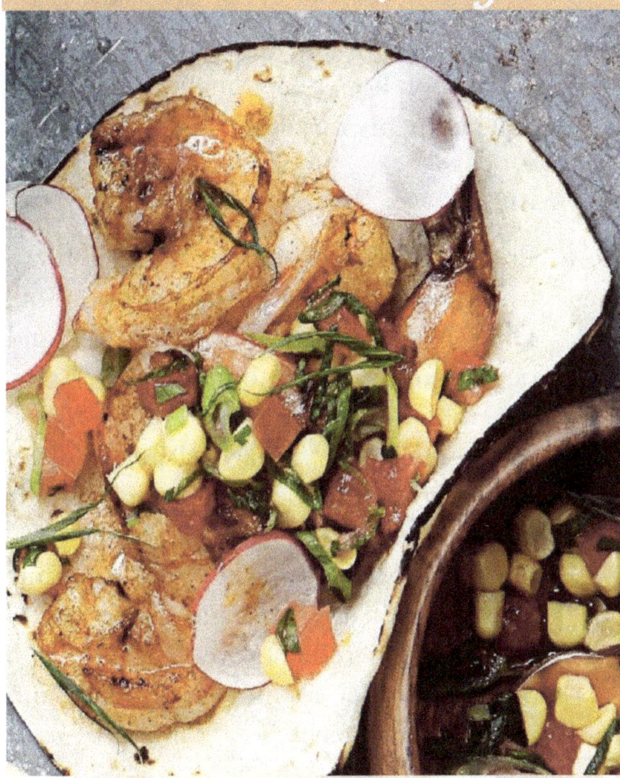

Preparation Time: 20 minutes

Ingredients:

- 1 lb large shrimp, peeled and deveined
- 1 tbsp olive oil
- 2 cloves garlic, minced
- 1 tsp chili powder
- 1 tsp cumin
- 1/2 tsp smoked paprika
- Juice of 1 lime
- Salt and pepper to taste
- 8 small lettuce leaves or almond flour tortillas
- 1 cup shredded red cabbage
- 1 avocado, sliced
- Fresh cilantro, chopped
- Salsa or pico de gallo (optional)

Procedure:

- In a medium bowl, combine the olive oil, garlic, chili powder, cumin, smoked paprika, lime juice, salt, and pepper.
- Add the shrimp to the bowl and toss to coat them evenly with the seasoning mixture. Let marinate for 10 minutes.
- Heat a large skillet over medium-high heat. Add the shrimp and cook for 2-3 minutes on each side, until they are pink and cooked through.
- Assemble the tacos by placing the cooked shrimp onto lettuce leaves or almond flour tortillas.
- Top with shredded red cabbage, avocado slices, fresh cilantro, and a spoonful of salsa or pico de gallo if desired.
- Serve immediately and enjoy your zesty shrimp tacos!

Nutritional Information (per serving):

- Calories: 250
- Protein: 20g
- Carbohydrates: 10g
- Fat: 15g
- Fiber: 4g
- Sugar: 2g

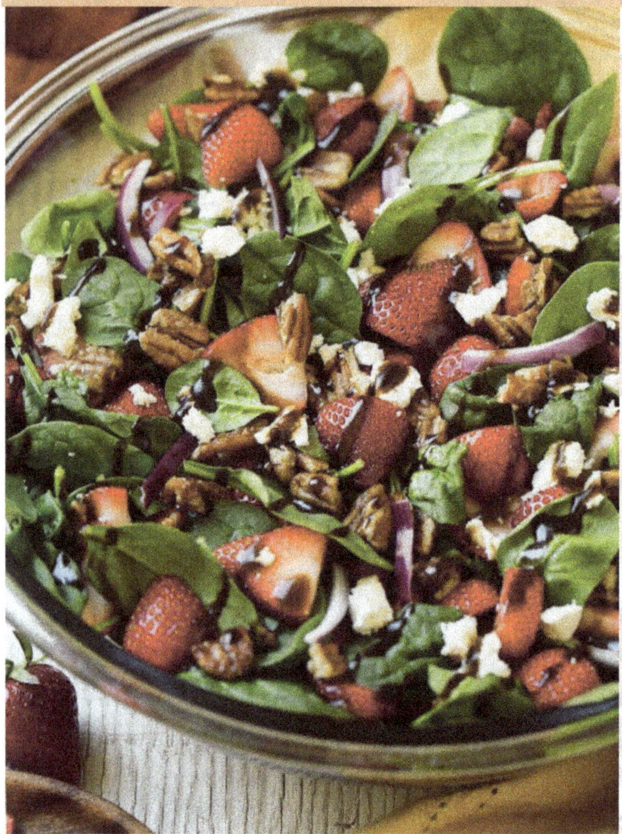

Ingredients:

- 4 cups fresh spinach leaves
- 1 cup strawberries, sliced
- 1/4 cup walnuts, chopped
- 1/4 cup red onion, thinly sliced
- 1/4 cup balsamic vinegar
- 2 tablespoons extra virgin olive oil
- 1 teaspoon Dijon mustard
- 1 teaspoon honey (optional)
- Salt and pepper to taste

Procedure:

- Prepare the Dressing: In a small bowl, whisk together balsamic vinegar, olive oil, Dijon mustard, honey (if using), salt, and pepper until well combined.
- Assemble the Salad: In a large bowl, combine fresh spinach leaves, sliced strawberries, chopped walnuts, and thinly sliced red onion.
- Dress the Salad: Drizzle the balsamic dressing over the salad and toss gently to coat all the ingredients evenly.
- Serve: Transfer to individual plates and serve immediately.

Nutritional Information (per serving, serves 4):

- Calories: 150
- Protein: 3g
- Carbohydrates: 10g
- Dietary Fiber: 3g
- Sugars: 6g
- Fat: 12g
- Saturated Fat: 1.5g
- Sodium: 75mg

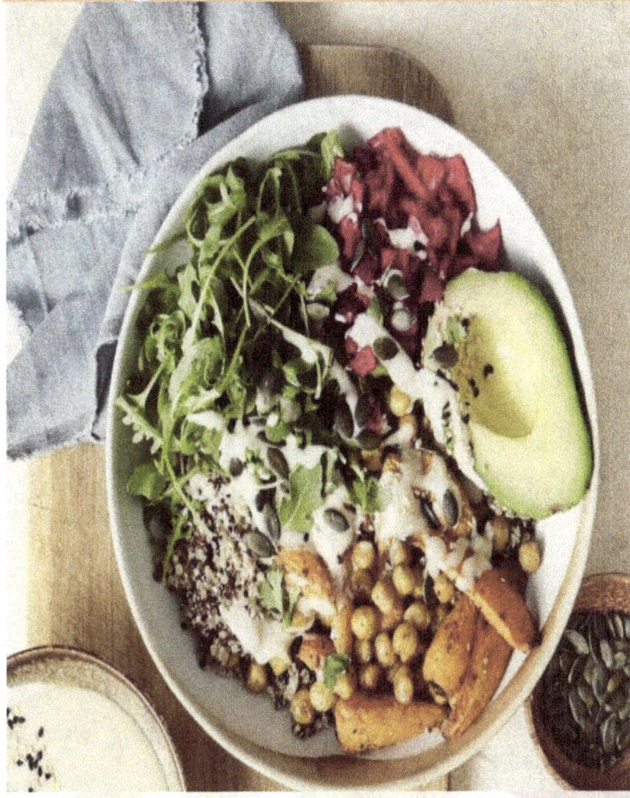

Preparation Time: 30 minutes

Ingredients:

- 1 cup quinoa, cooked
- 1 cup mixed greens (spinach, kale, arugula)
- 1 cup roasted vegetables (sweet potatoes, bell peppers, zucchini)
- 1/2 cup shredded carrots
- 1/2 avocado, sliced
- 1/4 cup chickpeas, cooked
- 2 tbsp pumpkin seeds
- 2 tbsp tahini
- 1 tbsp lemon juice
- 1 clove garlic, minced
- 2-3 tbsp water (to thin the dressing)
- Salt and pepper to taste

Procedure:

- Cook the Quinoa: Rinse 1 cup of quinoa under cold water. In a medium pot, combine quinoa with 2 cups of water and a pinch of salt. Bring to a boil, then reduce heat to low, cover, and simmer for 15 minutes until water is absorbed. Fluff with a fork.
- Roast the Vegetables: Preheat your oven to 400°F (200°C). Chop sweet potatoes, bell peppers, and zucchini into bite-sized pieces. Toss with a bit of olive oil, salt, and pepper. Spread on a baking sheet and roast for 20 minutes, stirring halfway through.
- Prepare the Dressing: In a small bowl, whisk together tahini, lemon juice, minced garlic, and water. Adjust the thickness by adding more water if necessary. Season with salt and pepper.
- Assemble the Bowl: In a large bowl, layer the cooked quinoa, mixed greens, roasted vegetables, shredded carrots, sliced avocado, and chickpeas. Sprinkle pumpkin seeds on top.
- Drizzle with Dressing: Pour the tahini dressing over the assembled bowl. Toss gently to combine all ingredients.

Nutritional Information (per serving):

- Calories: 450
- Protein: 15g
- Carbohydrates: 50g
- Fat: 22g
- Fiber: 12g
- Sugars: 6g

CHAPTER 6: PEGAN DINNER RECIPES

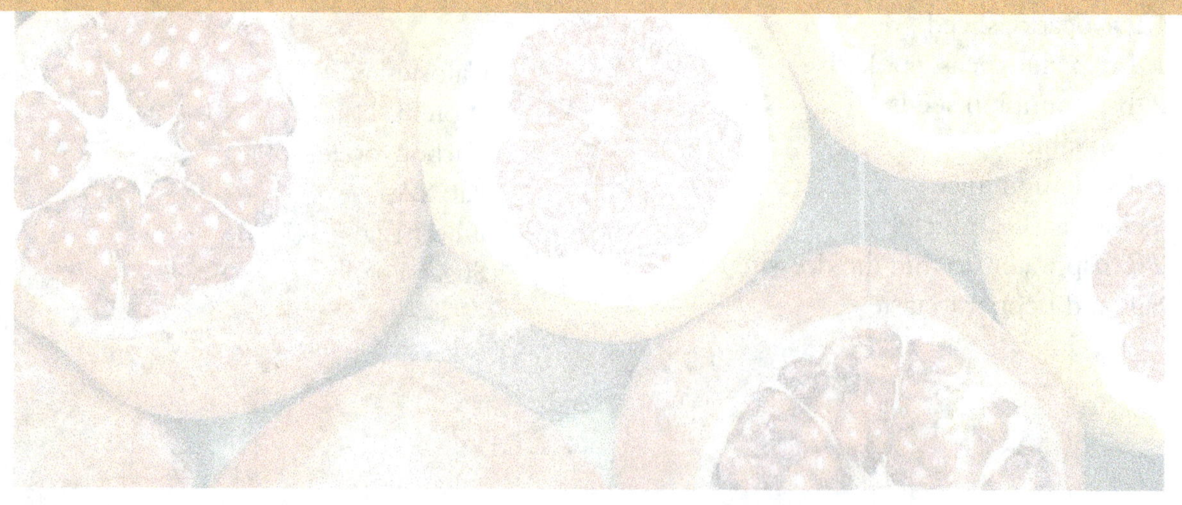

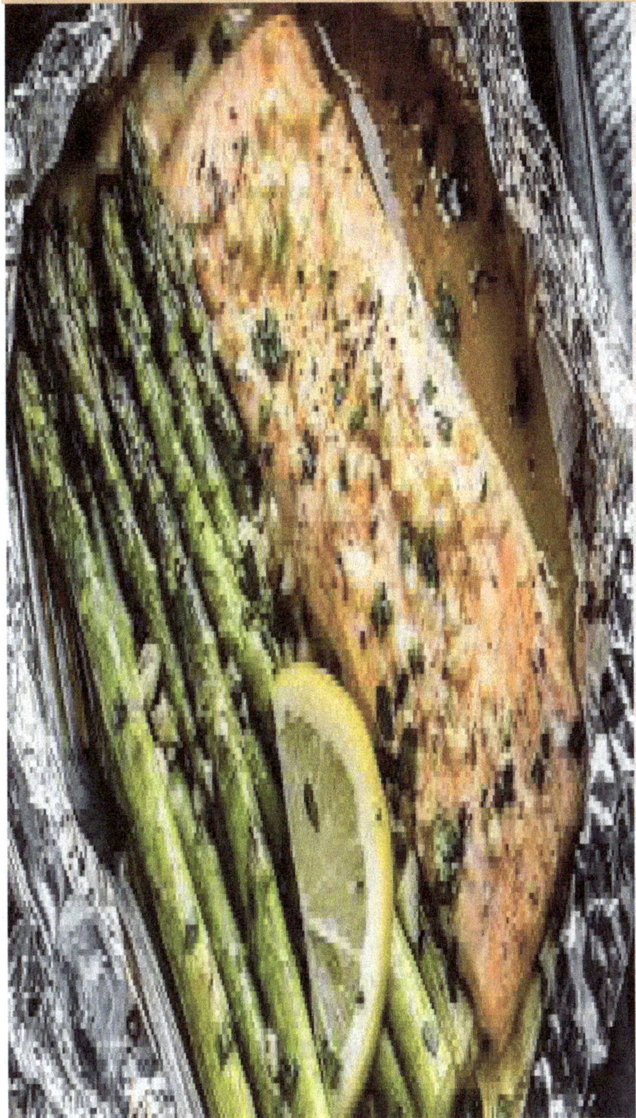

- 2 tablespoons olive oil
- 1 lemon, sliced
- 2 garlic cloves, minced
- Salt and pepper to taste
- Fresh dill for garnish

Procedure:

- Preheat your oven to 400°F (200°C).
- Place the salmon fillets and asparagus on a baking sheet lined with parchment paper.
- Drizzle olive oil over the salmon and asparagus.
- Sprinkle minced garlic, salt, and pepper evenly over everything.
- Arrange lemon slices on top of the salmon fillets.
- Bake in the preheated oven for 20 minutes or until the salmon is cooked through and flakes easily with a fork, and the asparagus is tender.
- Garnish with fresh dill before serving.

Nutritional Information (per serving):

- Calories: 350
- Protein: 30g
- Fat: 20g
- Carbohydrates: 6g
- Fiber: 3g
- Omega-3 fatty acids: High

Preparation Time: 30 minutes

Ingredients:

- 2 salmon fillets (6 oz each)
- 1 bunch of asparagus, trimmed

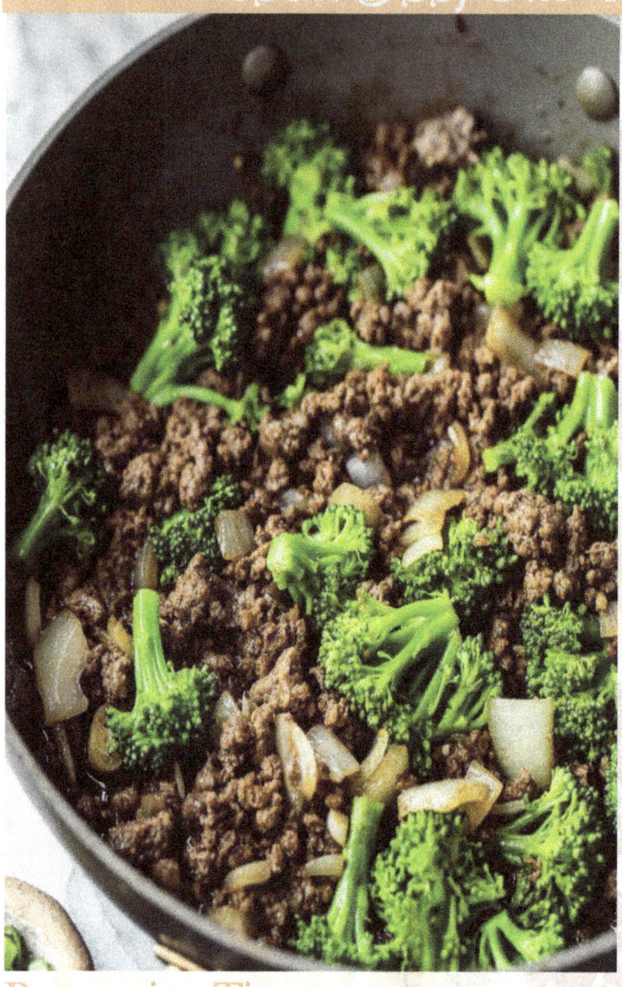

Preparation Time:
Total: 30 minutes
Prep: 15 minutes
Cook: 15 minutes

Ingredients:
- 1 lb lean beef, thinly sliced
- 2 cups broccoli florets
- 1 red bell pepper, sliced
- 1 small onion, sliced
- 3 cloves garlic, minced
- 2 tbsp coconut aminos (or tamari for a gluten-free option)
- 1 tbsp sesame oil
- 1 tbsp avocado oil
- 1 tsp fresh ginger, grated
- 1 tbsp sesame seeds (optional)
- Salt and pepper to taste

Procedure:
- Prepare the Ingredients: Thinly slice the beef and vegetables. Mince the garlic and grate the ginger.
- Heat the Pan: In a large skillet or wok, heat the avocado oil over medium-high heat.
- Cook the Beef: Add the beef to the hot skillet. Stir-fry for about 3-4 minutes until browned. Remove the beef from the skillet and set aside.
- Stir-Fry the Vegetables: In the same skillet, add the sesame oil. Add garlic and ginger, and sauté for about 30 seconds until fragrant. Add broccoli, bell pepper, and onion. Stir-fry for about 5-7 minutes until the vegetables are tender-crisp.
- Combine and Season: Return the beef to the skillet. Add coconut aminos (or tamari) and stir to combine. Cook for another 2-3 minutes until everything is heated through. Season with salt and pepper to taste.
- Garnish and Serve: Sprinkle with sesame seeds if desired. Serve hot.

Nutritional Information (per serving):
- Calories: 300
- Protein: 25g
- Carbohydrates: 10g
- Dietary Fiber: 3g
- Sugars: 4g
- Fat: 18g
- Saturated Fat: 4g
- Sodium: 400mg

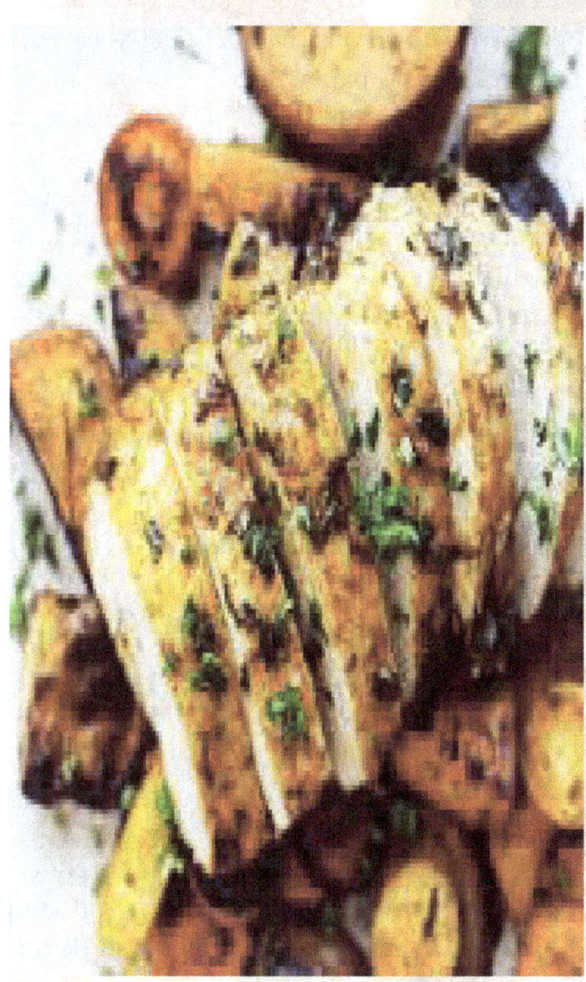

Preparation Time: 1 hour

Ingredients:

- 4 chicken thighs (bone-in, skin-on)
- 2 large sweet potatoes, peeled and cut into cubes
- 3 tablespoons olive oil
- 2 teaspoons dried rosemary
- 2 teaspoons dried thyme
- 2 garlic cloves, minced
- Salt and pepper to taste

Procedure:

- Preheat your oven to 400°F (200°C).
- In a large bowl, toss the sweet potato cubes with 1 tablespoon of olive oil, 1 teaspoon of rosemary, 1 teaspoon of thyme, and a pinch of salt and pepper. Spread the sweet potatoes on a baking sheet.
- In the same bowl, combine the chicken thighs with the remaining olive oil, rosemary, thyme, garlic, salt, and pepper. Rub the mixture evenly over the chicken.
- Place the chicken thighs on top of the sweet potatoes on the baking sheet.
- Roast in the preheated oven for about 45 minutes, or until the chicken is cooked through and the sweet potatoes are tender, stirring the potatoes halfway through.
- Serve hot, enjoying the delicious combination of herb-roasted chicken and caramelized sweet potatoes.

Nutritional Information (per serving):

- Calories: 450
- Protein: 28g
- Fat: 28g
- Carbohydrates: 20g
- Fiber: 4g
- Sugar: 5g

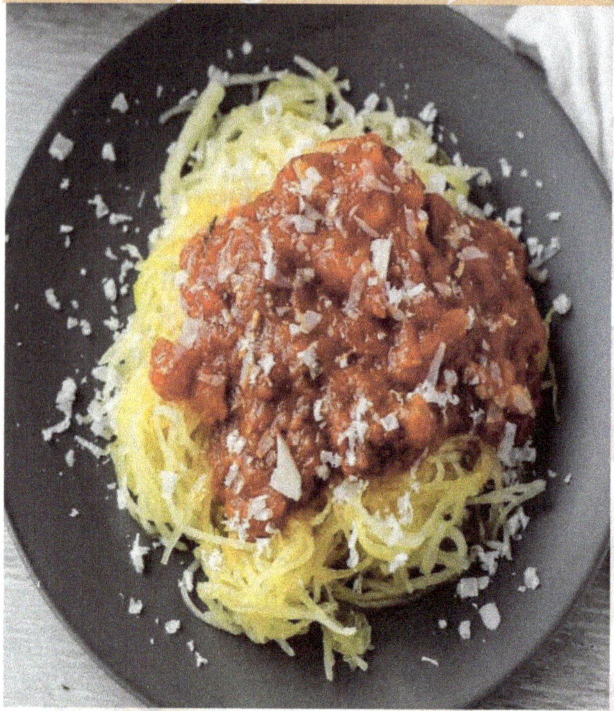

Preparation Time: 45 minutes

Ingredients:

- 1 large spaghetti squash
- 2 cups marinara sauce (preferably homemade or low-sugar, organic)
- 2 tablespoons olive oil
- 2 cloves garlic, minced
- 1 small onion, finely chopped
- 1 teaspoon dried oregano
- 1 teaspoon dried basil
- Salt and pepper to taste
- Fresh basil for garnish (optional)

Procedure:

- Preheat the Oven: Preheat your oven to 400°F (200°C).
- Prepare the Squash: Cut the spaghetti squash in half lengthwise and scoop out the seeds. Brush the inside with olive oil and season with salt and pepper.
- Bake the Squash: Place the squash halves cut-side down on a baking sheet lined with parchment paper. Bake for 35-40 minutes, or until the flesh is tender and easily shredded with a fork.
- Prepare the Sauce: While the squash is baking, heat the remaining olive oil in a large pan over medium heat. Add the chopped onion and garlic, sautéing until they are soft and fragrant.
- Simmer the Sauce: Add the marinara sauce, oregano, and basil to the pan. Stir well and let the sauce simmer on low heat for about 10-15 minutes, allowing the flavors to meld together. Season with salt and pepper to taste.
- Shred the Squash: Once the squash is cooked, remove it from the oven and let it cool slightly. Use a fork to scrape out the flesh, which will come out in spaghetti-like strands.

- Combine and Serve: Divide the shredded squash between plates and top with the marinara sauce. Garnish with fresh basil if desired.

Nutritional Information (per serving):

- Calories: 180
- Protein: 4g
- Carbohydrates: 25g
- Dietary Fiber: 6g
- Sugars: 10g
- Fat: 8g
- Saturated Fat: 1g
- Sodium: 400mg

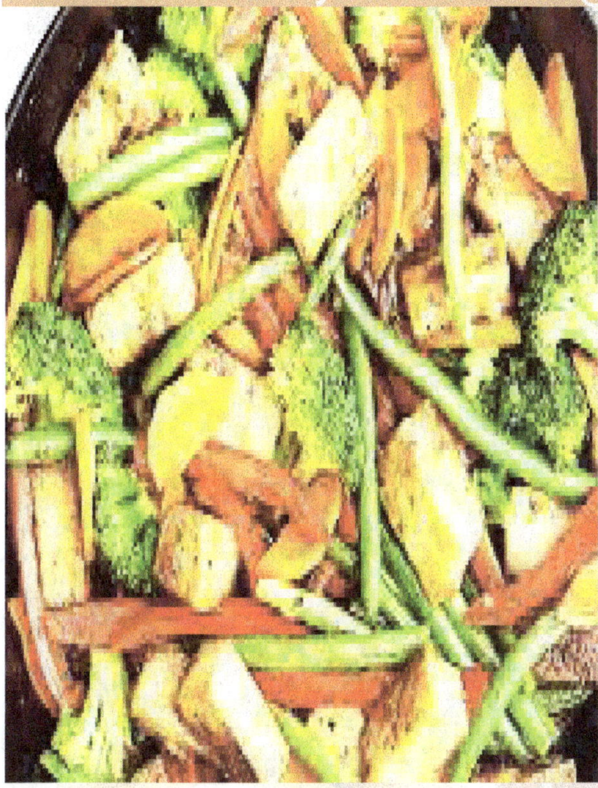

Preparation Time: 20 minutes

Ingredients:

* 1 block of firm tofu, pressed and cubed
* 2 tablespoons olive oil
* 1 bell pepper, sliced
* 1 zucchini, sliced
* 1 cup broccoli florets
* 1 carrot, julienned
* 2 cloves garlic, minced
* 1 tablespoon ginger, minced
* 2 tablespoons tamari or coconut aminos
* 1 tablespoon sesame oil
* 1 tablespoon sesame seeds (optional)
* Salt and pepper to taste

Procedure:

* Prepare the Tofu: Press the tofu to remove excess water, then cut it into cubes.
* Cook the Tofu: Heat 1 tablespoon of olive oil in a large skillet over medium-high heat. Add the tofu cubes and cook until golden brown on all sides, about 5-7 minutes. Remove tofu from skillet and set aside.
* Stir-Fry the Vegetables: In the same skillet, add the remaining olive oil. Add garlic and ginger, and sauté until fragrant, about 1 minute. Add bell pepper, zucchini, broccoli, and carrot. Stir-fry for 5-7 minutes until vegetables are tender-crisp.
* Combine and Season: Return the tofu to the skillet. Add tamari (or coconut aminos) and sesame oil, stirring to coat everything evenly. Cook for an additional 2-3 minutes.
* Finish and Serve: Season with salt and pepper to taste. Sprinkle with sesame seeds if desired. Serve hot.

Nutritional Information (Per Serving):

* Calories: 250
* Protein: 15g
* Carbohydrates: 12g
* Fiber: 5g
* Fat: 18g
* Vitamins and Minerals: Rich in Vitamin A, Vitamin C, calcium, and iron

CHAPTER 7: PEGAN DESSERT RECIPES

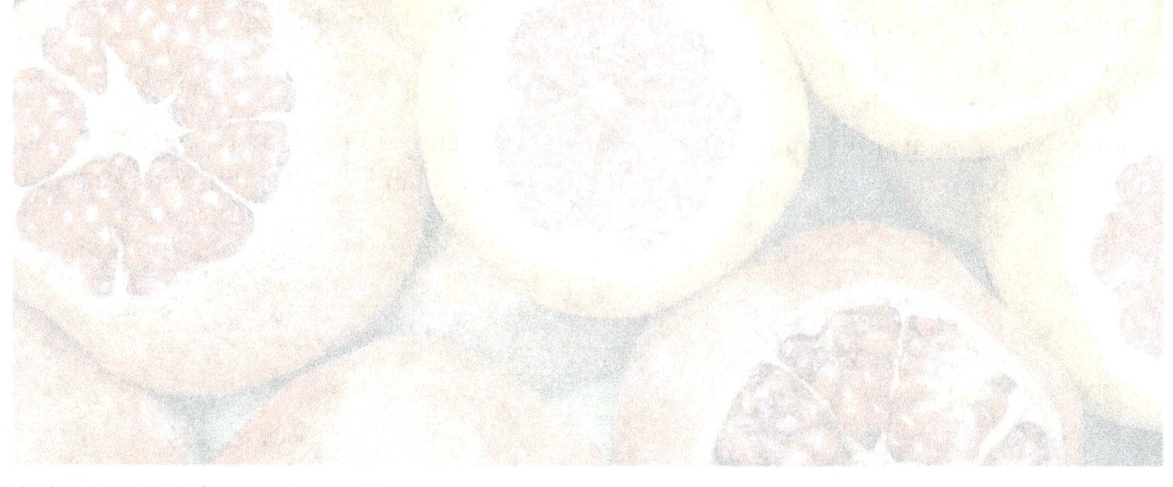

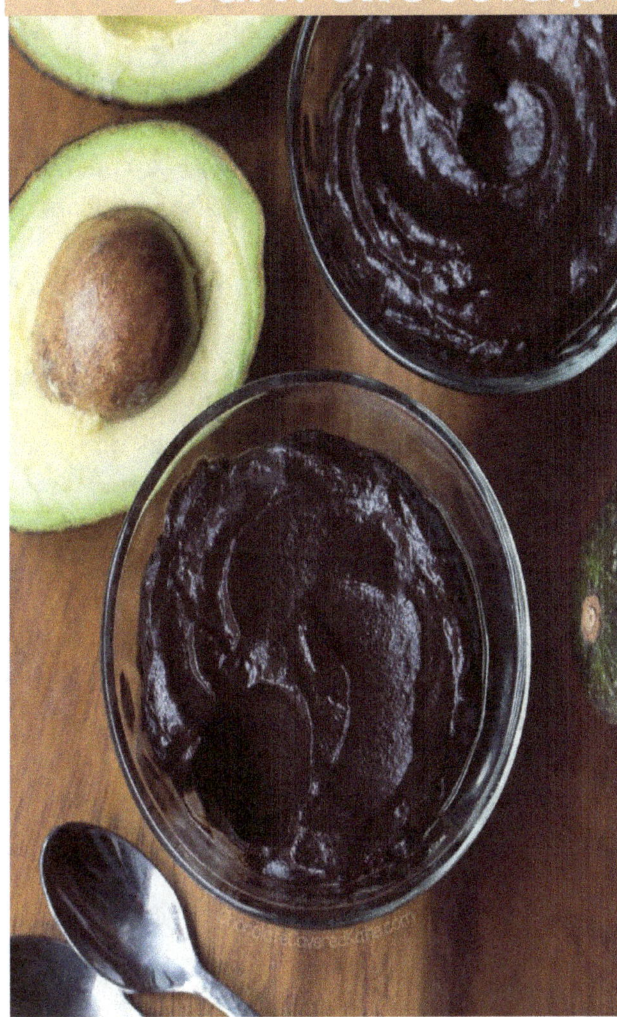

* 1/4 cup pure maple syrup
* 1/4 cup coconut milk (full-fat)
* 1 tsp vanilla extract
* A pinch of sea salt

Procedure:

* **Blend Ingredients:** In a food processor or blender, combine the avocados, cocoa powder, maple syrup, coconut milk, vanilla extract, and sea salt. Blend until smooth and creamy.
* **Adjust Sweetness:** Taste the mousse and adjust sweetness, if desired, by adding more maple syrup.
* **Chill:** Transfer the mousse to serving bowls and refrigerate for at least 1 hour to let the flavors meld and the texture set.
* **Serve:** Garnish with fresh berries or a sprinkle of cocoa powder before serving, if desired.

Nutritional Information (per serving, makes 4 servings):

* Calories: 180
* Protein: 2 g
* Fat: 12 g
* Carbohydrates: 20 g
* Fiber: 5 g
* Sugar: 12 g

Preparation Time: 10 minutes
Chilling Time: 1 hour

Ingredients:

* 2 ripe avocados
* 1/4 cup unsweetened cocoa powder

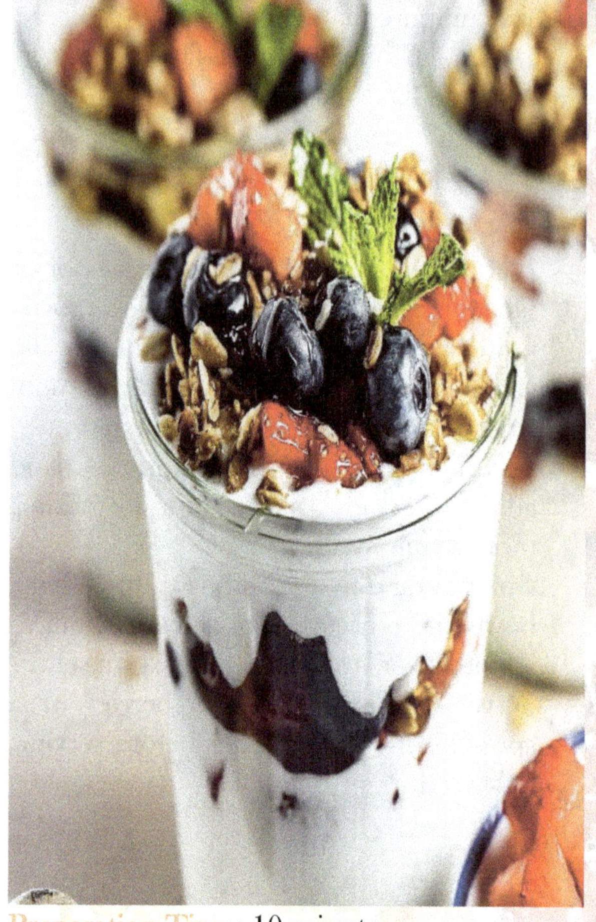

Preparation Time: 10 minutes

Ingredients:

- 1 cup plain Greek yogurt
- 1/2 cup mixed fresh berries (strawberries, blueberries, raspberries)
- 1/4 cup granola (Pegan-friendly)
- 1 tablespoon chia seeds
- 1 tablespoon honey (optional)

Procedure:

- Layer the Yogurt: Spoon 1/4 cup of Greek yogurt into the bottom of a serving glass or bowl.
- Add Berries: Top the yogurt with a layer of fresh berries.
- Sprinkle Granola: Add a layer of granola over the berries.
- Chia Seeds: Sprinkle chia seeds on top of the granola.
- Repeat Layers: Repeat the layers with the remaining yogurt, berries, granola, and chia seeds.
- Finish with Honey: Drizzle a small amount of honey over the top if desired.
- Serve Immediately: Enjoy the parfait fresh, or refrigerate for up to 2 hours before serving.

Nutritional Information (per serving):

- Calories: 250
- Protein: 14g
- Fat: 7g
- Carbohydrates: 30g
- Fiber: 6g
- Sugars: 15g

Almond Flour Brownies

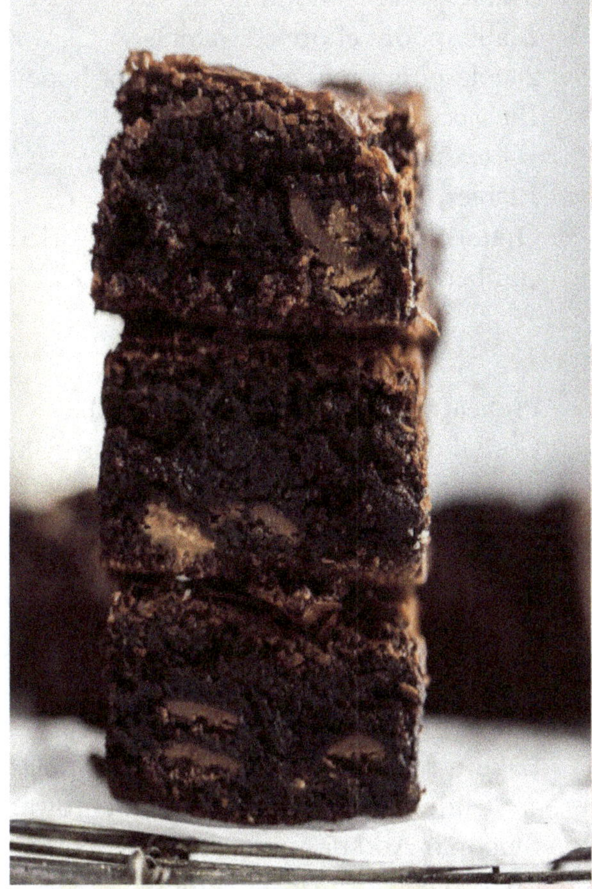

Preparation Time: 15 minutes
Cooking Time: 25 minutes
Total Time: 40 minutes

Ingredients:

- 1 cup almond flour
- 1/2 cup unsweetened cocoa powder
- 1/4 cup maple syrup
- 1/4 cup coconut oil (melted)
- 2 large eggs
- 1/4 cup coconut sugar
- 1 teaspoon vanilla extract
- 1/4 teaspoon sea salt
- 1/2 teaspoon baking powder

Procedure:

- **Preheat Oven:** Set your oven to 350°F (175°C) and line an 8x8-inch baking pan with parchment paper.
- **Mix Dry Ingredients:** In a large bowl, whisk together almond flour, cocoa powder, coconut sugar, baking powder, and sea salt.
- **Combine Wet Ingredients:** In another bowl, beat the eggs, then stir in the maple syrup, melted coconut oil, and vanilla extract.
- **Combine Mixtures:** Gradually add the wet ingredients to the dry ingredients, mixing until well combined.
- **Bake:** Pour the batter into the prepared pan and smooth the top with a spatula. Bake for 20-25 minutes, or until a toothpick inserted into the center comes out mostly clean.
- **Cool and Slice:** Let the brownies cool in the pan before slicing into squares.

Nutritional Information (per serving, based on 9 servings):

- Calories: 180
- Protein: 4g
- Carbohydrates: 15g
- Fiber: 3g
- Sugar: 8g
- Fat: 12g
- Saturated Fat: 4g

Baked Apple with Cinnamon

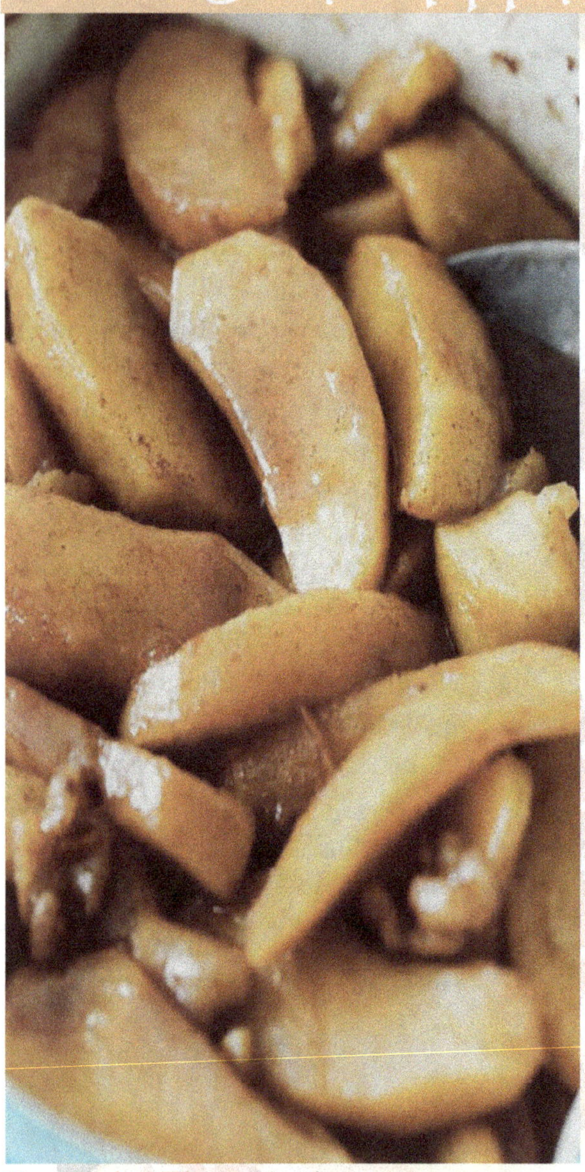

- 2 tablespoons almond flour
- 2 tablespoons chopped walnuts
- 2 tablespoons pure maple syrup or honey
- 1 teaspoon ground cinnamon
- 1/4 teaspoon ground nutmeg
- 1 tablespoon coconut oil (melted)
- Optional: 1 tablespoon raisins or dried cranberries

Procedure:

- Preheat your oven to 350°F (175°C).
- Core the apples, creating a small cavity in the center of each.
- In a small bowl, mix almond flour, chopped walnuts, cinnamon, nutmeg, and maple syrup or honey.
- Stuff the apple cavities with the mixture.
- Place the apples in a baking dish and drizzle with melted coconut oil.
- Bake for 30 minutes, or until the apples are tender and the filling is golden brown.
- Optional: Add raisins or dried cranberries to the filling for extra sweetness.

Nutritional Information (per serving, assuming 4 apples):

- Calories: 150
- Protein: 2 g
- Fat: 6 g
- Carbohydrates: 24 g
- Fiber: 4 g
- Sugars: 16 g

Preparation Time: 10 minutes
Cooking Time: 30 minutes
Total Time: 40 minutes

Ingredients:

- 4 medium apples (such as Gala or Fuji)

Preparation Time: 10 minutes (plus 4 hours chilling)

Ingredients:

- 1/4 cup chia seeds
- 1 cup almond milk (or any Pegan-approved plant-based milk)
- 1 tablespoon maple syrup (or honey for a non-vegan option)
- 1/2 teaspoon vanilla extract
- 1/2 cup mixed berries (such as strawberries, blueberries, and raspberries)

Procedure:

- Combine Ingredients: In a medium bowl, mix chia seeds, almond milk, maple syrup, and vanilla extract until well combined.
- Chill: Cover the bowl and refrigerate for at least 4 hours, or overnight. Stir the mixture occasionally to prevent clumping.
- Serve: Once the pudding has thickened, stir it well and divide it into serving bowls. Top with mixed berries before serving.

Nutritional Information (per serving):

- Calories: 150
- Protein: 4g
- Fat: 8g
- Carbohydrates: 15g
- Fiber: 8g
- Sugar: 7g

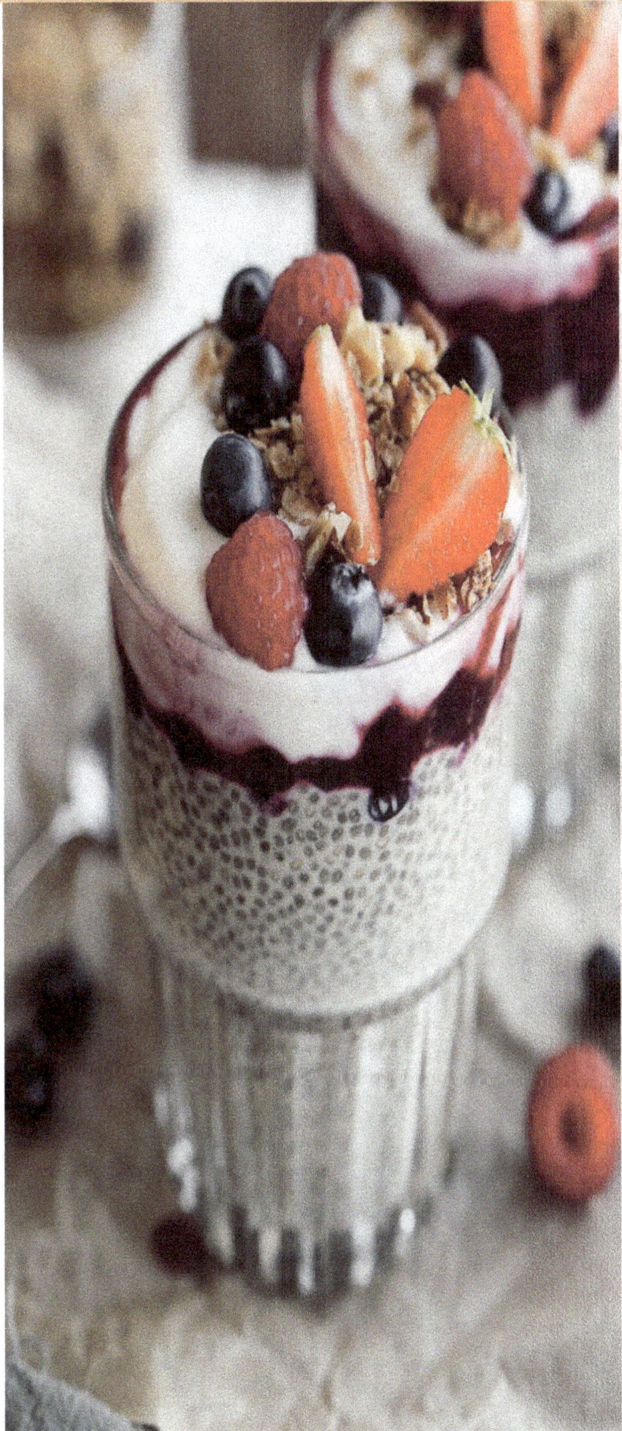

CHAPTER 8: PEGAN SNACKS AND APPETIZERS

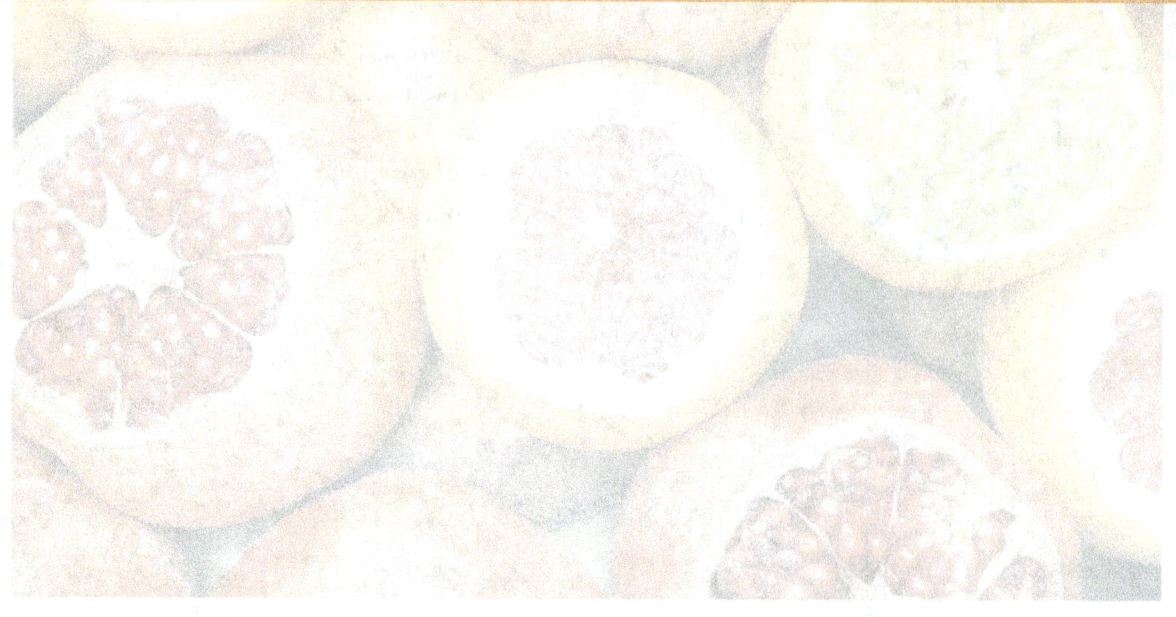

- 1/2 teaspoon sea salt
- 1/4 teaspoon black pepper
- 1/4 teaspoon cayenne pepper (optional, for heat)

Procedure:

- Preheat your oven to 350°F (175°C) and line a baking sheet with parchment paper.
- In a large bowl, combine all nuts and seeds.
- Drizzle with olive oil and toss to coat evenly.
- Sprinkle smoked paprika, ground cumin, garlic powder, onion powder, sea salt, black pepper, and cayenne pepper (if using) over the nuts and seeds. Toss again to ensure an even coating of the spices.
- Spread the mixture in a single layer on the prepared baking sheet.
- Roast in the oven for 12-15 minutes, stirring halfway through, until nuts are golden and fragrant.
- Allow to cool completely before serving or storing.

Nutritional Information (per 1/4 cup serving):

- Calories: 180
- Protein: 6g
- Fat: 16g
- Saturated Fat: 1.5g
- Carbohydrates: 7g
- Dietary Fiber: 3g
- Sugars: 1g
- Sodium: 150mg

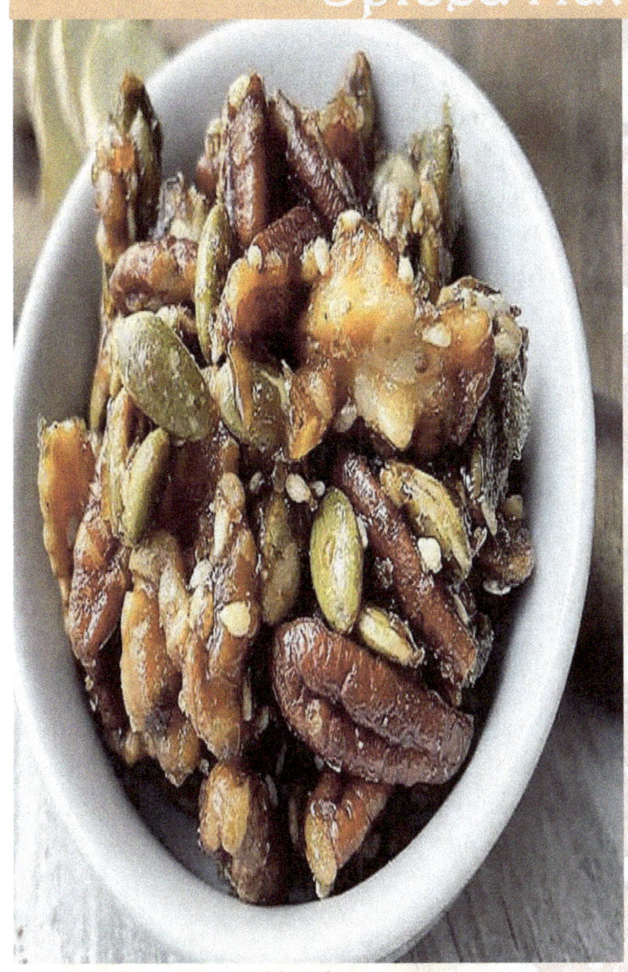

Preparation Time: 10 minutes
Cooking Time: 15 minutes
Total Time: 25 minutes

Ingredients:

- 1 cup raw almonds
- 1 cup raw cashews
- 1/2 cup raw pumpkin seeds
- 1/2 cup raw sunflower seeds
- 2 tablespoons olive oil
- 1 teaspoon smoked paprika
- 1 teaspoon ground cumin
- 1/2 teaspoon garlic powder
- 1/2 teaspoon onion powder

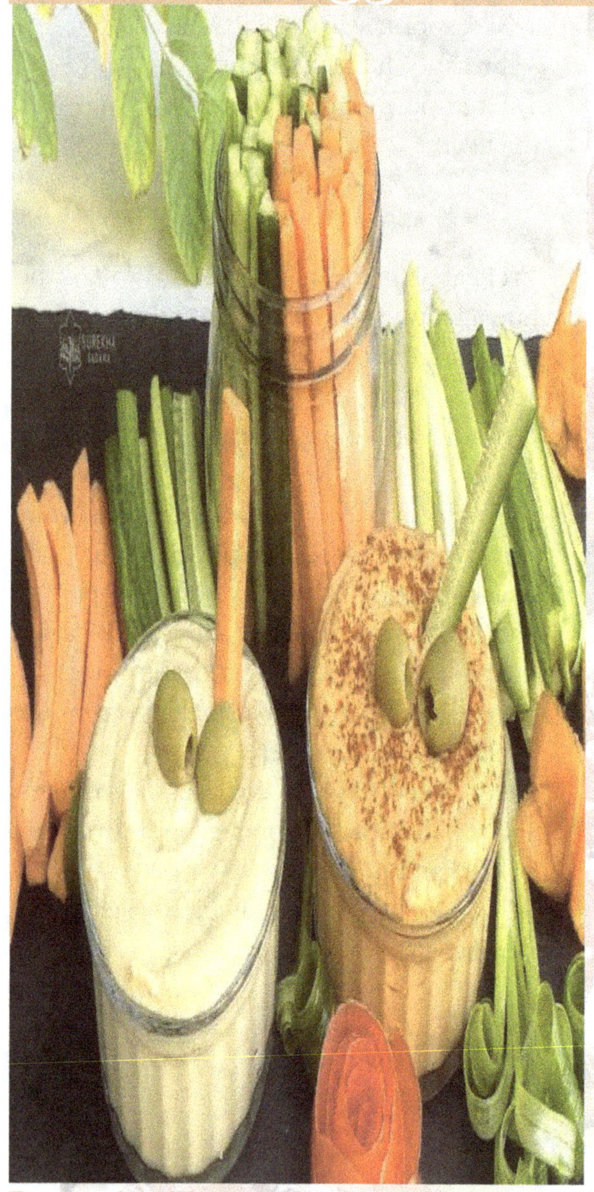

*   1 cup of baby carrots
*   1 cup of cucumber sticks
*   1 cup of bell pepper strips (any color)
*   1 cup of celery sticks
*   1 cup of cherry tomatoes
*   1 cup of hummus (store-bought or homemade)

Procedure:

*   Prepare the Vegetables: Wash and peel the baby carrots. Slice the cucumbers, bell peppers, and celery into sticks. Cut the cherry tomatoes in half if preferred.
*   Arrange the Veggies: Place all the prepared vegetable sticks and cherry tomatoes on a serving platter or individual plates.
*   Serve with Hummus: Scoop the hummus into a small bowl and place it in the center of the platter or next to the veggies for dipping.

Nutritional Information (per serving):

*   Calories: 150
*   Protein: 5g
*   Fat: 8g
*   Carbohydrates: 18g
*   Fiber: 5g
*   Sugars: 6g

Preparation Time: 15 minutes

Ingredients:

Pegan Energy Bars

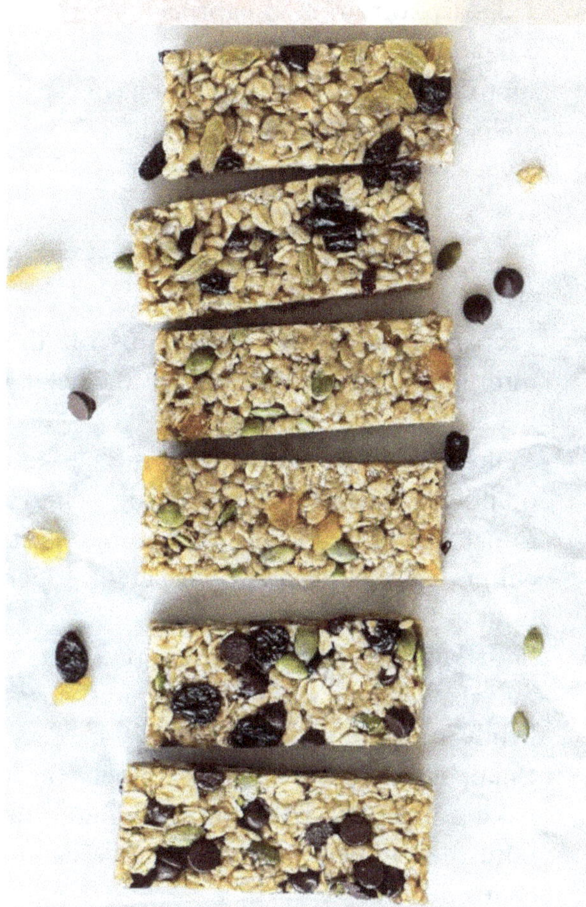

Preparation Time: 15 minutes
Chilling Time: 1 hour
Makes: 12 bars

Ingredients:

- 1 cup pitted dates
- 1 cup raw nuts (such as almonds or cashews)
- 1/2 cup shredded coconut
- 1/4 cup chia seeds
- 1/4 cup unsweetened cocoa powder
- 2 tablespoons almond butter
- 1 tablespoon honey or maple syrup (optional, for added sweetness)

Procedure:

- Prep the Dates: Place pitted dates in a food processor and blend until they form a sticky paste.
- Process the Nuts: Add the raw nuts to the processor and pulse until finely chopped but not pulverized.
- Combine Ingredients: Add shredded coconut, chia seeds, cocoa powder, and almond butter to the mixture. Blend until everything is well combined.
- Sweeten (Optional): If using, add honey or maple syrup and blend again.
- Press Mixture: Transfer the mixture to an 8x8-inch baking dish lined with parchment paper. Press it down firmly and evenly with a spatula.
- Chill: Refrigerate for at least 1 hour to firm up.
- Cut and Serve: Once set, lift the mixture out of the dish using the parchment paper, cut into bars, and serve.

Nutritional Information (per bar):

- Calories: 180
- Protein: 4g
- Fat: 12g
- Carbohydrates: 15g
- Fiber: 3g
- Sugar: 8g

Stuffed Mini Peppers

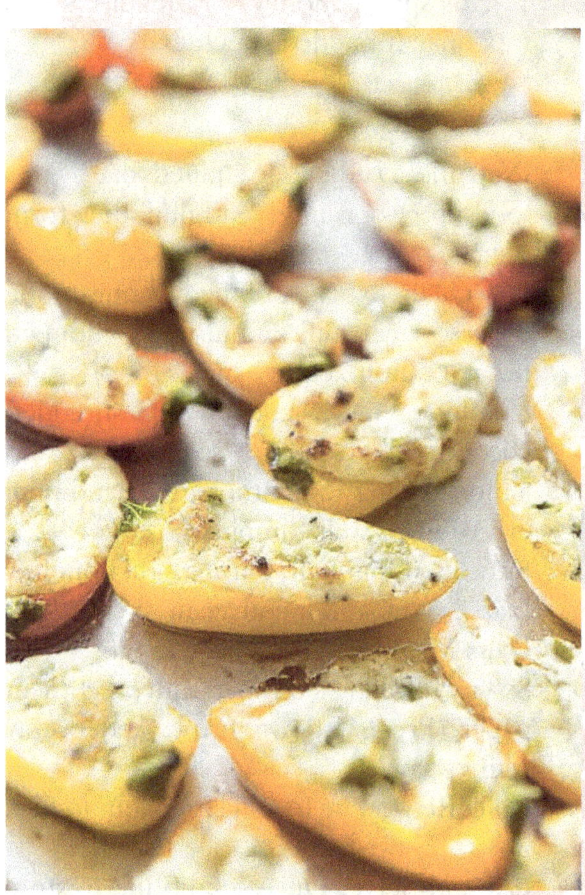

Preparation Time: 20 minutes
Cooking Time: 15 minutes
Total Time: 35 minutes

Ingredients:

- 12 mini bell peppers
- 1 cup cooked quinoa
- 1/2 cup black beans, drained and rinsed
- 1/2 cup corn kernels (fresh or frozen)
- 1/2 cup cherry tomatoes, diced
- 1/4 cup red onion, finely chopped
- 2 tablespoons fresh cilantro, chopped
- 1 tablespoon olive oil
- 1 teaspoon cumin
- 1/2 teaspoon smoked paprika
- Salt and pepper to taste
- Optional: 1/4 cup crumbled feta cheese (if including dairy in your Pegan diet)

Procedure:

- Preheat Oven: Preheat your oven to 375°F (190°C).
- Prepare Peppers: Slice the tops off the mini bell peppers and remove the seeds. Set aside.
- Make Filling: In a bowl, mix the cooked quinoa, black beans, corn, cherry tomatoes, red onion, cilantro, olive oil, cumin, smoked paprika, salt, and pepper until well combined.
- Stuff Peppers: Spoon the quinoa mixture into each mini pepper, pressing down lightly to pack the filling.
- Bake: Arrange the stuffed peppers on a baking sheet and bake for 15 minutes, or until the peppers are tender and slightly charred.
- Optional Cheese: If using feta cheese, sprinkle it on top of the peppers during the last 5 minutes of baking.

Nutritional Information (per serving, 2 stuffed peppers):

- Calories: 150
- Protein: 5g
- Carbohydrates: 20g
- Fat: 7g
- Fiber: 4g
- Sugars: 5g

Kale Chips

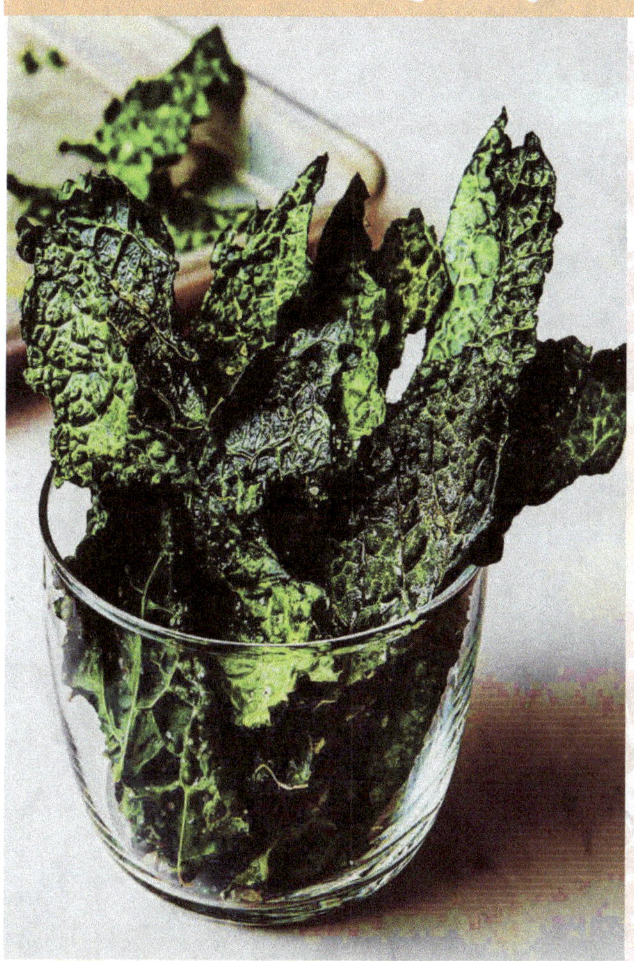

Ingredients:

- 1 bunch of kale (about 8-10 large leaves)
- 1-2 tablespoons olive oil
- 1/2 teaspoon sea salt
- 1/2 teaspoon garlic powder (optional)
- 1/2 teaspoon paprika (optional)

Procedure:

- **Preheat Oven:** Set your oven to 350°F (175°C).
- **Prepare Kale:** Wash the kale leaves thoroughly and pat them dry with a clean towel. Remove the tough stems and tear the leaves into bite-sized pieces.
- **Season Kale:** In a large bowl, toss the kale leaves with olive oil, ensuring each piece is lightly coated. Sprinkle with sea salt, and add garlic powder and paprika if desired.
- **Bake:** Spread the kale pieces evenly on a baking sheet lined with parchment paper. Bake for 10-15 minutes, or until the edges are crisp and the leaves are crunchy. Be sure to check frequently to prevent burning.
- **Cool and Serve:** Let the kale chips cool on the baking sheet for a few minutes before serving. Enjoy as a healthy snack or a crunchy salad topping.

Nutritional Information (per serving, about 1 cup):

- Calories: 70
- Protein: 2g
- Fat: 5g
- Saturated Fat: 0.5g
- Carbohydrates: 6g
- Fiber: 2g
- Sugars: 1g
- Sodium: 150mg

CHAPTER 9: PEGAN DRINKS AND SMOOTHIES

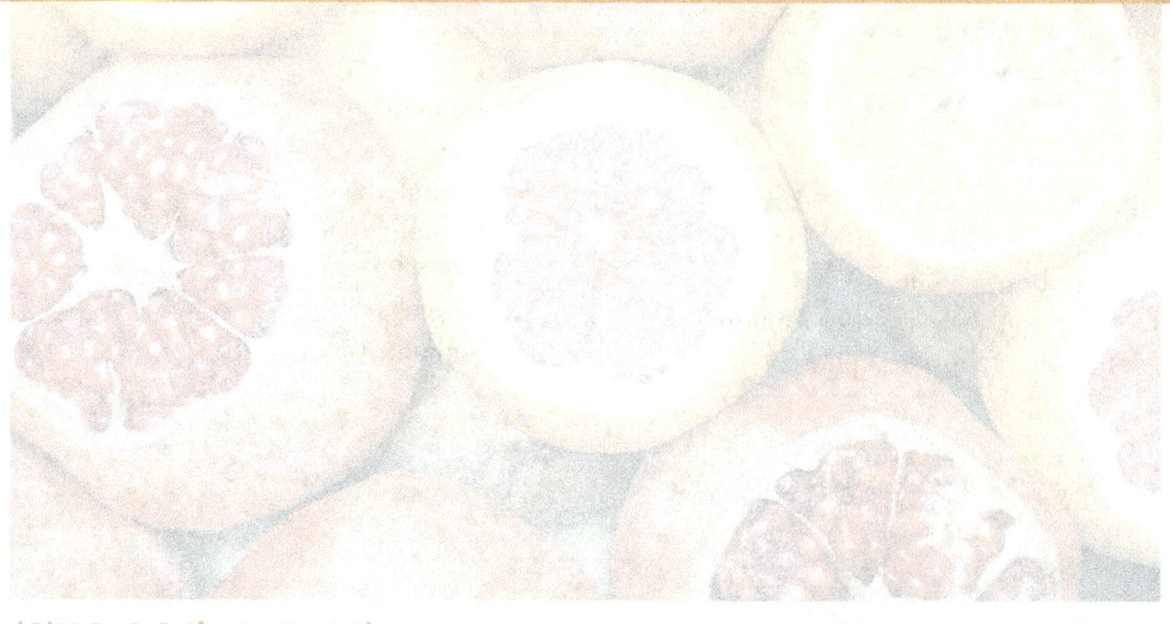

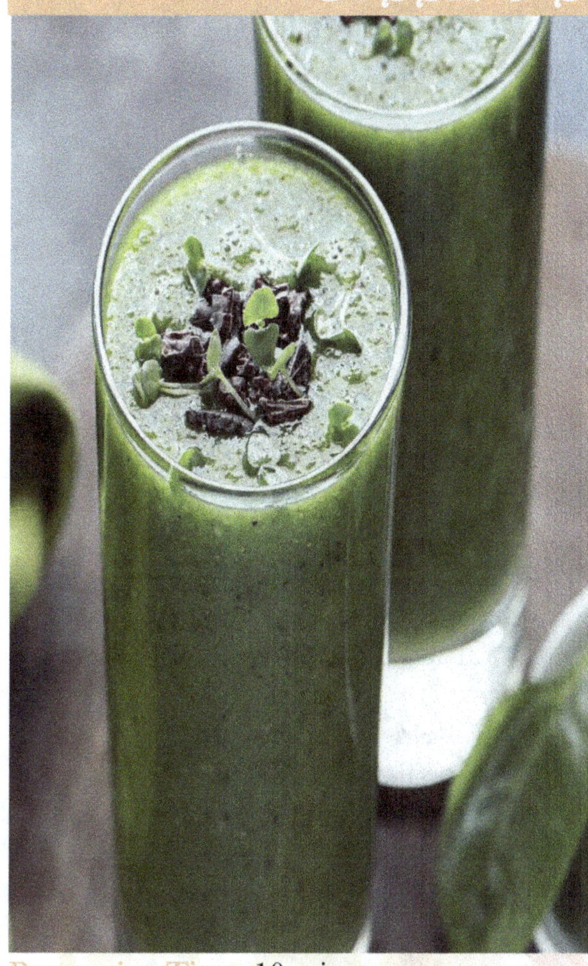

Preparation Time: 10 minutes

Ingredients:

- 1 cup spinach leaves
- 1/2 cup kale, stems removed
- 1 green apple, cored and chopped
- 1/2 cucumber, peeled and sliced
- 1/2 lemon, juiced
- 1 tablespoon chia seeds
- 1 cup unsweetened almond milk (or other plant-based milk)
- 1/2 inch fresh ginger, peeled
- Ice cubes (optional)

Procedure:

- In a blender, combine the spinach, kale, apple, cucumber, and ginger.
- Add the lemon juice, chia seeds, and almond milk.
- Blend on high until smooth. If desired, add ice cubes for a chilled smoothie.
- Pour into a glass and serve immediately for the best flavor and nutrient retention.

Nutritional Information (per serving):

- Calories: 150
- Protein: 3 grams
- Fat: 4 grams
- Carbohydrates: 30 grams
- Fiber: 6 grams
- Sugar: 14 grams
- Vitamin A: 130% DV
- Vitamin C: 60% DV
- Calcium: 20% DV
- Iron: 15% DV

Preparation Time: 5 minutes

Ingredients:

- 1 lemon, sliced
- A handful of fresh mint leaves
- 4 cups of filtered water
- Ice cubes (optional)

Procedure:

- Prepare Ingredients: Wash the lemon and mint leaves thoroughly. Slice the lemon into thin rounds.
- Combine: In a large pitcher, add the lemon slices and fresh mint leaves.
- Infuse: Pour the filtered water over the lemon and mint. Stir gently to release the flavors.
- Chill: Refrigerate for at least 2 hours to allow the flavors to infuse. Add ice cubes if desired before serving.

Nutritional Information (per 1 cup serving):

- Calories: 0
- Total Fat: 0g
- Sodium: 0mg
- Total Carbohydrates: 0g
- Sugars: 0g
- Protein: 0g

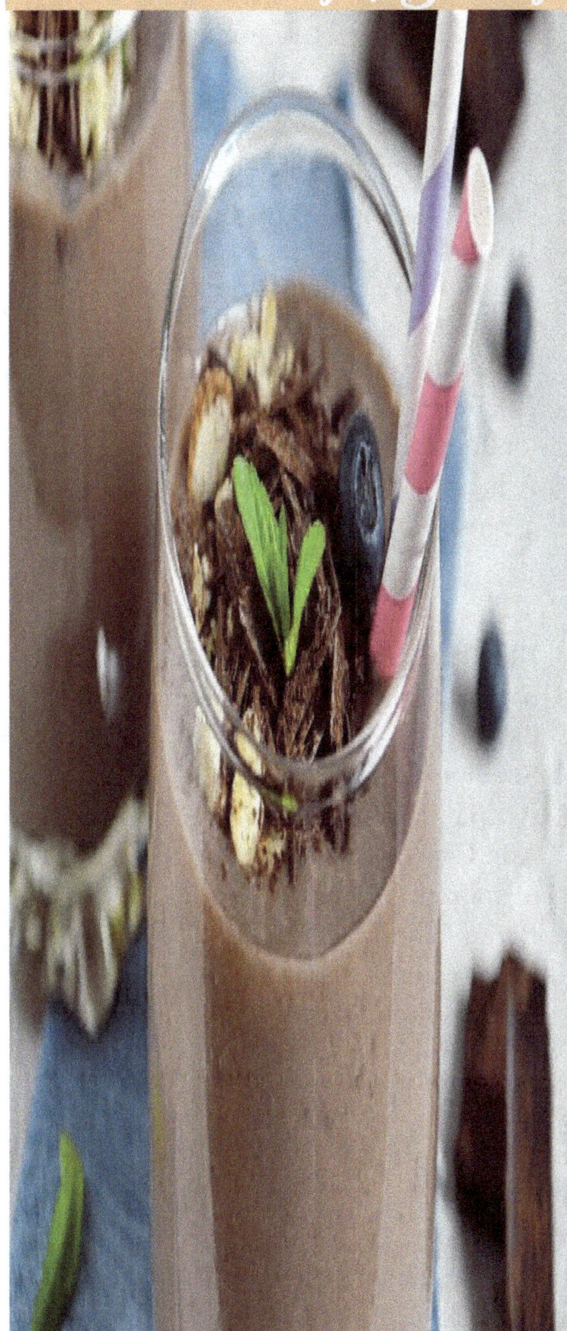

Ingredients:

- 1 cup unsweetened almond milk
- 1 scoop plant-based protein powder (pea, hemp, or brown rice)
- 1 banana
- 1 tablespoon chia seeds
- 1 tablespoon almond butter
- 1 cup spinach leaves
- 1/2 cup frozen berries (such as blueberries or strawberries)
- Optional: 1 teaspoon honey or maple syrup for sweetness

Procedure:

- Add the almond milk, plant-based protein powder, banana, chia seeds, and almond butter to a blender.
- Toss in the spinach leaves and frozen berries.
- Blend on high until smooth and creamy.
- Taste and adjust sweetness with honey or maple syrup if desired.
- Pour into a glass and enjoy immediately.

Nutritional Information (per serving):

- Calories: 320
- Protein: 20g
- Carbohydrates: 35g
- Fats: 12g
- Fiber: 8g
- Sugar: 15g (natural sugars from fruit and optional sweetener)

Preparation Time: 5 minutes

Berry Blast Smoothie

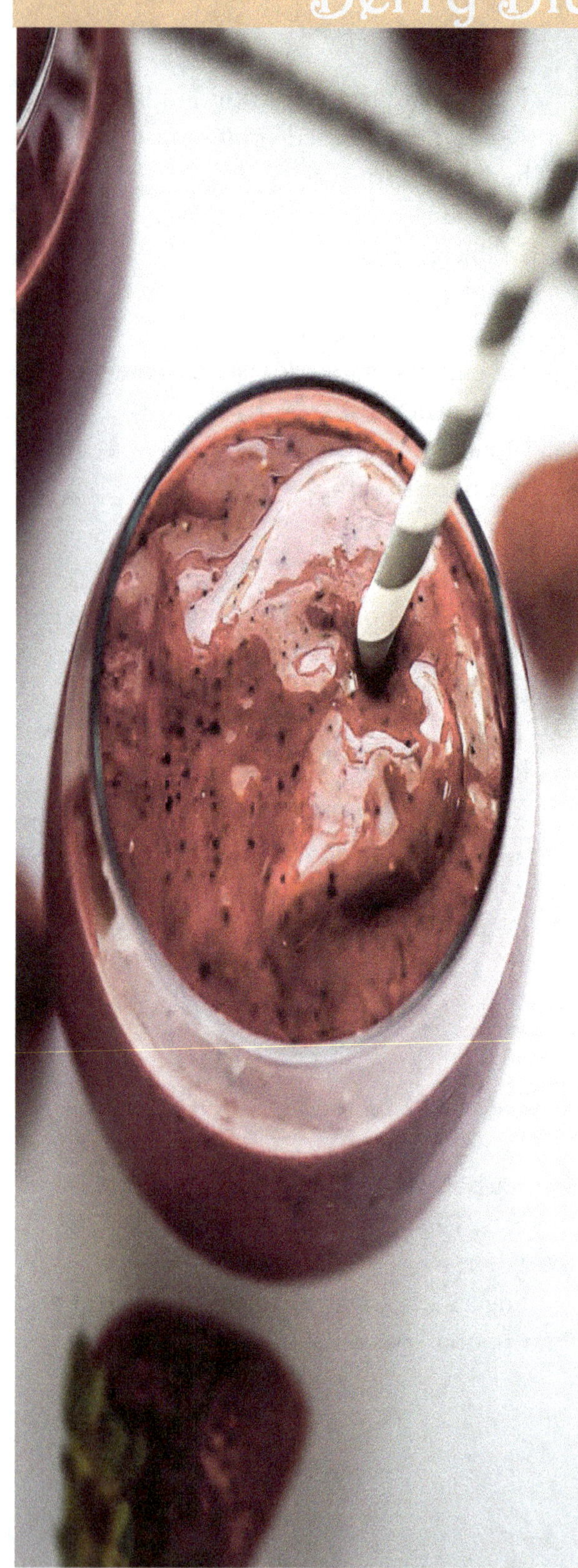

Preparation Time: 10 minutes

Ingredients:

- 1 cup mixed berries (strawberries, blueberries, raspberries)
- 1 banana
- 1 cup unsweetened almond milk (or any Pegan-friendly milk)
- 1 tablespoon chia seeds
- 1 tablespoon honey or maple syrup (optional, for added sweetness)
- A handful of spinach (optional, for extra greens)

Procedure:

- Blend: Combine the mixed berries, banana, almond milk, and chia seeds in a blender.
- Sweeten (Optional): Add honey or maple syrup if desired for extra sweetness.
- Add Greens (Optional): Toss in a handful of spinach for a nutrient boost.
- Blend Thoroughly: Blend until smooth and creamy.
- Serve: Pour into a glass and enjoy immediately for the best flavor and texture.

Nutritional Information (per serving):

- Calories: 200
- Protein: 4g
- Carbohydrates: 34g
- Dietary Fiber: 8g
- Sugars: 20g
- Fat: 6g
- Vitamin C: 80% of Daily Value
- Calcium: 20% of Daily Value

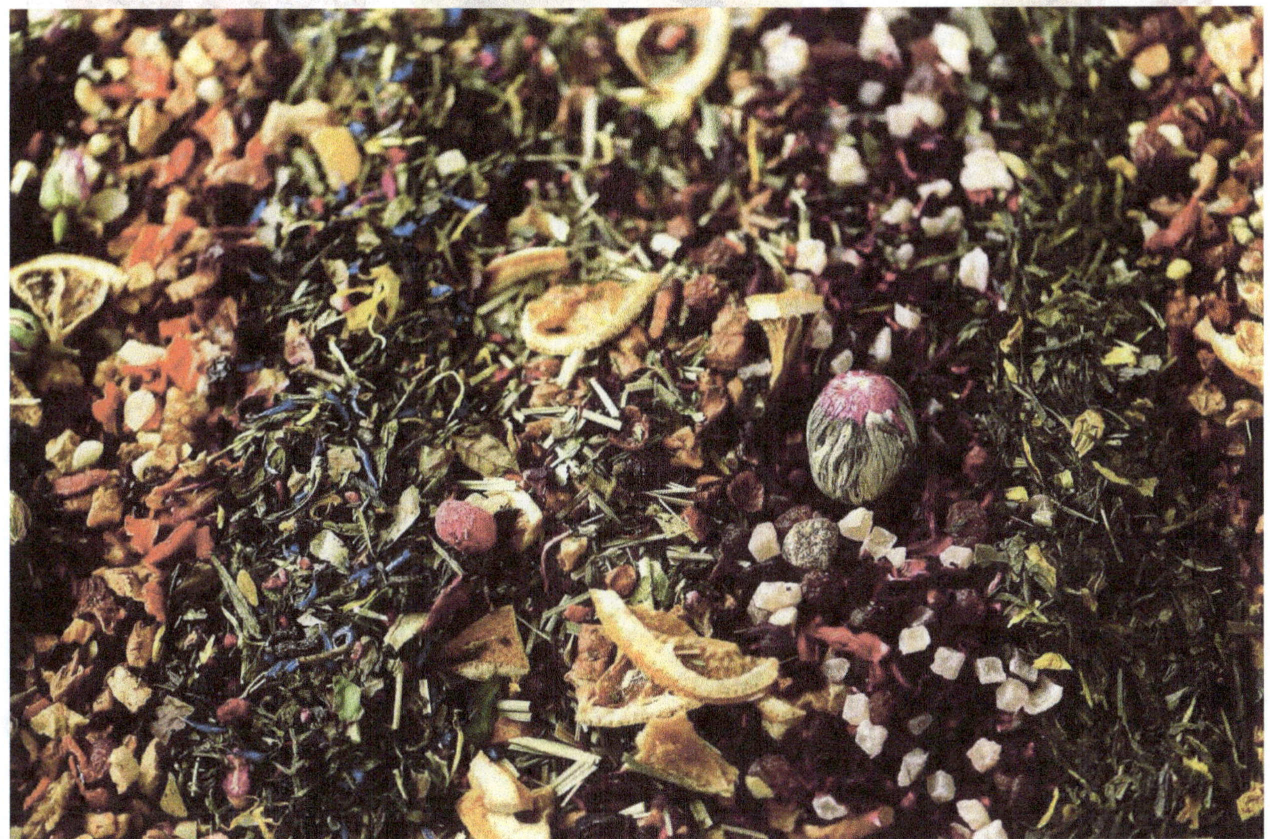

Herbal teas are a delightful and soothing way to enhance your Pegan diet, offering a range of health benefits and complementing a wholesome, plant-based lifestyle. Rich in antioxidants and beneficial compounds, these teas can support digestion, boost immunity, and provide relaxation.

Preparation Time: 5-10 minutes

Ingredients:

- 1 herbal tea bag or 1 tablespoon of loose herbal tea (e.g., chamomile, peppermint, ginger, or rooibos)
- 1 cup of boiling water
- Optional: a slice of lemon or a teaspoon of honey

Procedure:

- **Boil Water:** Heat water until it reaches a rolling boil.
- **Steep Tea:** Place the herbal tea bag or loose tea in a cup. Pour the boiling water over the tea and let it steep for 5-7 minutes.

❖ **Add Extras:** If desired, add a slice of lemon or a teaspoon of honey for extra flavor.

❖ **Enjoy:** Remove the tea bag or strain out the loose tea. Sip and enjoy your soothing herbal tea.

Nutritional Information:

❖ **Calories**: 0-5 (depending on added ingredients)

❖ **Vitamins & Minerals**: Varies by herbal type. For example, chamomile can support relaxation, peppermint aids digestion, ginger offers anti-inflammatory properties, and rooibos is rich in antioxidants.

Health Benefits: Herbal teas can help reduce stress, improve digestion, support immune function, and provide a calming effect.

CHAPTER 10: PEGAN LIFESTYLE TIPS

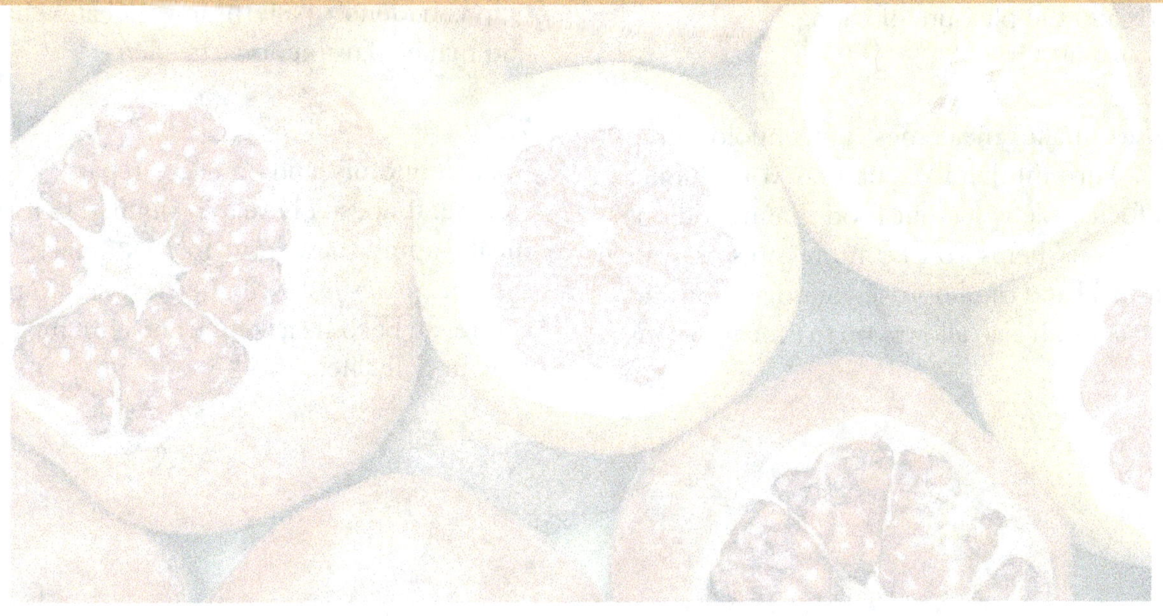

In a world where meals often become a matter of convenience rather than enjoyment, mindful eating stands as a refreshing antidote. It's not just about what you eat but how you eat, focusing your attention on the present moment and creating a deeper connection with your food.

1. Savor Each Bite

Start by taking a moment to appreciate the look, smell, and texture of your meal before you even take a bite. Notice the colors on your plate, the aroma wafting up, and the texture of the food. As you eat, chew slowly and savor each bite. This not only enhances the taste experience but also helps you recognize when you're full, reducing the likelihood of overeating.

2. Engage All Your Senses

Mindful eating involves engaging all your senses. Feel the temperature of your food, listen to the crunch of a fresh vegetable, and enjoy the complex flavors as they unfold in your mouth. By fully engaging your senses, you become more attuned to your body's needs and the pleasure of eating.

3. Eat Without Distractions

Try to make mealtimes a technology-free zone. Turn off the TV, put away your phone, and focus solely on your food. Eating without distractions helps you be more present with your meal and can improve your digestion and satisfaction. It also allows you to tune into your body's hunger and fullness cues more effectively.

4. Listen to Your Body

Pay attention to how your body responds to different foods. Notice how you feel after eating—do you feel energized or sluggish? Do certain foods leave you feeling satisfied or still hungry? Listening to your body's signals can help you make more informed choices about what and how much to eat.

5. Practice Gratitude

Before diving into your meal, take a moment to express gratitude for the food on your plate. Acknowledge the effort it took to bring this food to your table, from the farmers who grew it to the cooks who prepared it. This practice not only enriches your eating experience but also fosters a positive relationship with food.

6. Reflect on Your Eating Habits

After your meal, spend a few moments reflecting on the experience. How did you feel during and after eating? Were you able to eat slowly and enjoy your food? Reflection can help you identify patterns in your eating habits and make adjustments as needed.

7. Incorporate Mindful Eating Into Daily Life

Make mindful eating a regular part of your routine. It doesn't have to be limited to formal meals—apply these principles to snacks and smaller meals as well. Over time, mindful eating can become a natural and enriching part of your daily life.

Embracing the Pegan lifestyle is about more than just what's on your plate—it's a holistic approach to well-being that extends to how you move and engage with your body. Staying active is a vital part of this journey, helping to balance the nourishing foods you eat with physical vitality. Here's how you can stay active and align your fitness routine with Pegan principles:

1. Find Activities You Love

Staying active doesn't mean you have to hit the gym every day or run marathons. The key is to find physical activities that bring you joy. Whether it's hiking through nature, dancing, practicing yoga, or swimming, the best exercise is the one you look forward to. Your passion for the activity will make it easier to stick with your routine.

2. Integrate Movement into Your Daily Life

Incorporating movement into your daily routine doesn't always require a structured workout. Simple changes, like taking the stairs instead of the elevator, going for a walk during your lunch break, or engaging in active hobbies like gardening, can significantly increase your daily activity levels. Every bit of movement counts and contributes to your overall well-being.

3. Combine Strength and Cardio

A balanced fitness routine should include both strength training and cardiovascular exercises. Strength training helps build lean muscle, which supports your metabolism and overall strength. Activities like resistance exercises, bodyweight workouts, or weightlifting can be paired with cardio exercises such as jogging, cycling, or brisk walking. This combination will help keep your body strong and your heart healthy.

4. Listen to Your Body

One of the core principles of Peganism is tuning into your body's needs. This extends to your fitness routine as well. Pay attention to how your body feels before, during, and after exercise. If you're tired or sore, allow yourself time to rest and recover. Overtraining can lead to injury and burnout, so balance your workouts with adequate rest.

5. Set Realistic Goals

Setting achievable goals can keep you motivated and focused. Start with small, realistic targets that align with your current fitness level and gradually increase them as you progress. Celebrate your milestones, no matter how small they may seem. This positive reinforcement helps maintain motivation and commitment to your fitness journey.

6. Make It Social

Exercise can be more enjoyable when shared with others. Join a local sports team, attend fitness classes, or find a workout buddy. Social interactions during physical activities can enhance your motivation and make the experience more enjoyable. Plus, having a support system can help you stay accountable to your fitness goals.

7. Mind-Body Connection

Integrate practices that enhance the mind-body connection, such as mindfulness, meditation, or deep breathing exercises. These practices can reduce stress and improve your overall mental well-being, which in turn supports a more balanced and effective physical fitness routine.

8. Stay Consistent

Consistency is key in any fitness routine. Aim to incorporate physical activity into your daily life regularly. Whether it's a short morning stretch, a midday walk, or an evening workout, maintaining a consistent routine will yield the best results over time.

9. Reflect and Adjust

Regularly reflect on your activity levels and how they fit with your Pegan lifestyle. Adjust your routine as needed to ensure it continues to meet your personal needs and goals. If you find that certain activities no longer resonate with you, don't hesitate to explore new forms of exercise.

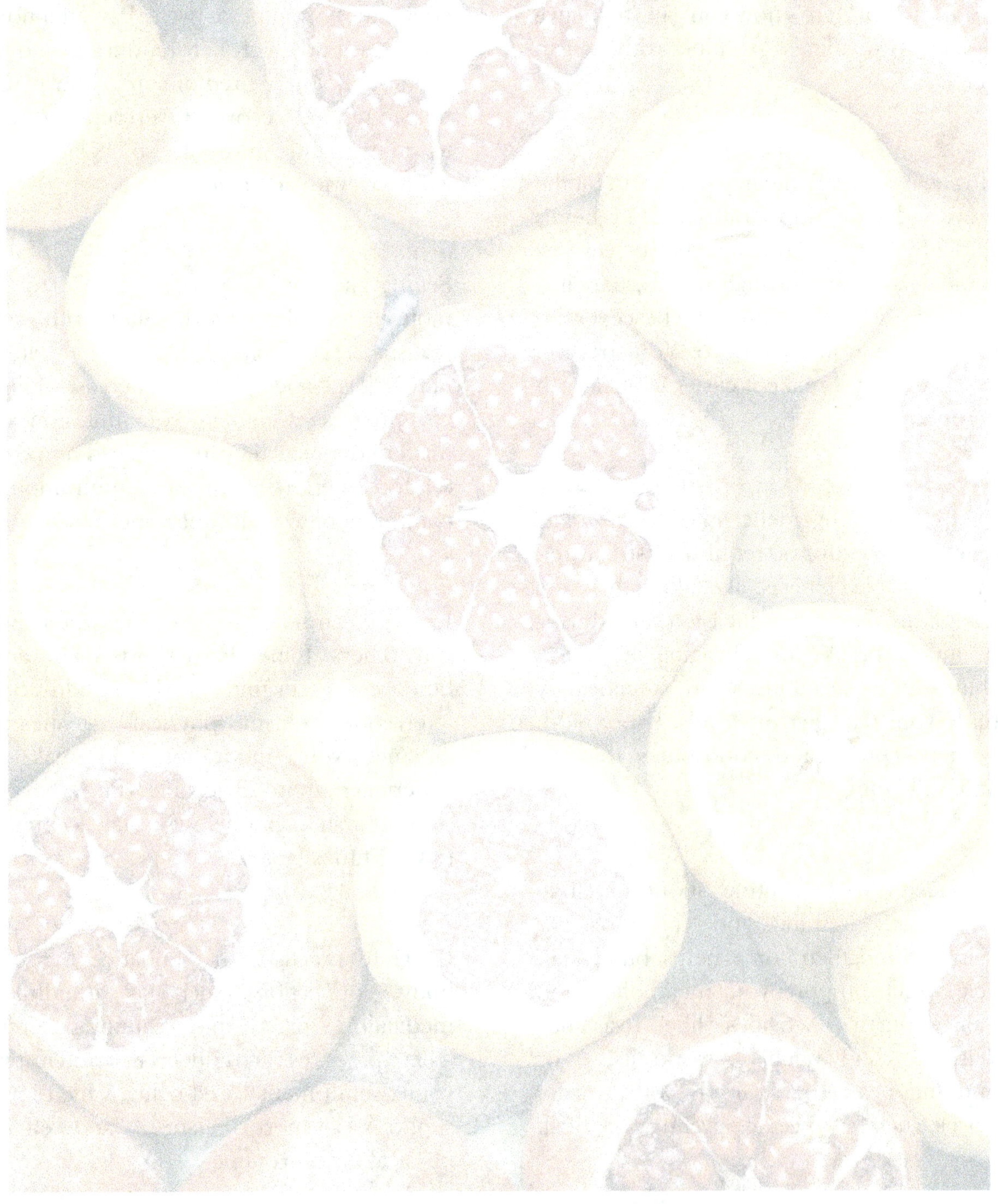

In today's fast-paced world, stress seems almost inevitable. From tight deadlines and personal responsibilities to unforeseen challenges, stress can creep into every corner of our lives. However, managing stress isn't just about surviving—it's about thriving and finding balance that leads to better health and overall well-being.

Understanding Stress and Its Impact

Stress is the body's natural response to perceived threats or challenges. It triggers a cascade of physiological reactions designed to help us deal with immediate dangers—what's often called the "fight-or-flight" response. While this reaction can be life-saving in short bursts, chronic stress can have a detrimental effect on our health. Prolonged stress can lead to headaches, fatigue, digestive problems, and even heart disease. Emotionally, it can cause anxiety, depression, and irritability.

Identifying Your Stressors

The first step in managing stress is understanding what causes it. Stressors vary widely from person to person. For some, it may be work-related pressures or financial worries. For others, it could be relationship issues or health concerns. By identifying your specific stressors, you can begin to address them more effectively. Keeping a journal of your daily stressors and noting your reactions can help in pinpointing patterns and triggers.

Practicing Mindfulness and Relaxation

Mindfulness is the practice of being fully present in the moment, without judgment. It can be a powerful tool in managing stress. Techniques such as meditation, deep breathing exercises, and progressive muscle relaxation can help calm the mind and reduce the body's stress response. Even a few minutes a day can make a significant difference. Apps and guided sessions can be helpful for beginners and can provide structure to your practice.

Maintaining a Healthy Lifestyle

A balanced diet, regular exercise, and adequate sleep are crucial in managing stress. Physical activity releases endorphins, the body's natural mood lifters, and helps reduce tension. Aim for at least 30 minutes of moderate exercise most days of the week. Eating a diet rich in fruits, vegetables, lean proteins, and whole grains provides the nutrients needed to cope with stress. And don't underestimate the power of sleep— quality rest is essential for both physical and mental health.

Building Strong Relationships

Having a support system of friends, family, or colleagues can make a huge difference in how you handle stress. Sharing your feelings with someone you trust can provide relief and perspective. Social connections not only offer emotional support but can also be a source of practical help in times of need.

Setting Boundaries and Managing Time

One common source of stress is feeling overwhelmed by responsibilities. Learning to set boundaries and manage your time effectively can help alleviate this. Prioritize tasks and focus on what's most important. Delegate where possible and don't be afraid to say no to additional commitments that may overwhelm you. Time management techniques, such as creating a daily schedule or breaking tasks into manageable steps, can also reduce stress.

Finding Joy and Relaxation

Incorporating activities that bring joy and relaxation into your routine is essential. Whether it's pursuing a hobby, spending time in nature, reading a book, or simply enjoying a warm bath, these moments of relaxation can recharge your batteries and provide a break from stressors.

Seeking Professional Help

Sometimes, stress can become overwhelming and difficult to manage on your own. If you find that stress is affecting your daily life or mental health, seeking help from a mental health professional is a positive step. Therapy can offer strategies for coping with stress, and sometimes just talking about your experiences can be immensely therapeutic.

Embracing a Positive Mindset

Finally, adopting a positive mindset can greatly influence how you handle stress. Focus on what you can control and practice gratitude for the positive aspects of your life. Small changes in perspective can make a significant impact on your stress levels and overall health.

Embracing the Pegan diet can be a transformative journey, not just for your health but for your overall well-being. One of the most enriching aspects of this lifestyle is the community that can grow around it. A supportive Pegan community doesn't just help you stay motivated and informed—it fosters a sense of belonging and shared purpose. Here's how you can build and nurture a supportive Pegan community.

1. Find Like-Minded Individuals
Start by connecting with others who share your Pegan values and goals. This might be through online forums, social media groups, or local meet-ups. Platforms like Facebook, Reddit, or dedicated Pegan forums can be great starting points. Look for groups that focus on Peganism or related interests such as plant-based nutrition, sustainable eating, or holistic health.

2. Share Your Journey
Openly sharing your experiences, challenges, and successes can help you build connections with others. Whether you're blogging about your Pegan journey, posting on social media, or participating in discussion groups, your stories can inspire and engage others. Sharing recipes, meal plans, and tips not only contributes to the community but can also invite feedback and encouragement.

3. Attend Events and Workshops
Participate in or organize events like cooking classes, health workshops, or Pegan potlucks. These gatherings provide opportunities for face-to-face interactions, which can strengthen bonds and deepen relationships. They also allow you to learn from experts, exchange ideas, and experience new recipes together.

4. Support Local Pegan Businesses
Supporting local Pegan-friendly businesses, such as health food stores, restaurants, or farmers' markets, helps create a network of like-minded entrepreneurs and advocates. These businesses often have their own communities and events that can offer additional support and resources.

5. Create a Support System
Form a small support group with friends or family who are interested in Peganism. Regular meetings, whether virtual or in person, can be a space for discussing experiences, sharing recipes, and offering encouragement. This support system can be crucial during challenging times or when facing new dietary hurdles.

6. Volunteer and Give Back
Engage with community outreach programs or charitable organizations that align with Pegan principles. Volunteering for causes related to nutrition, environmental sustainability, or animal welfare not only supports the broader mission of Peganism but also connects you with others who are passionate about making a positive impact.

7. Educate and Empower
Be a resource for others who are new to the Pegan diet. Offer to help friends and family understand the principles of Peganism, share beginner tips, or introduce them to Pegan-friendly recipes. Education fosters a sense of community and encourages others to embark on their own Pegan journeys.

8. Practice Inclusivity and Respect
A supportive community thrives on inclusivity and respect. Encourage open dialogue,

respect diverse perspectives, and support others in their personal Pegan journeys, even if their approach differs from yours. Acknowledging and celebrating these differences can strengthen the community and make it more welcoming to everyone.

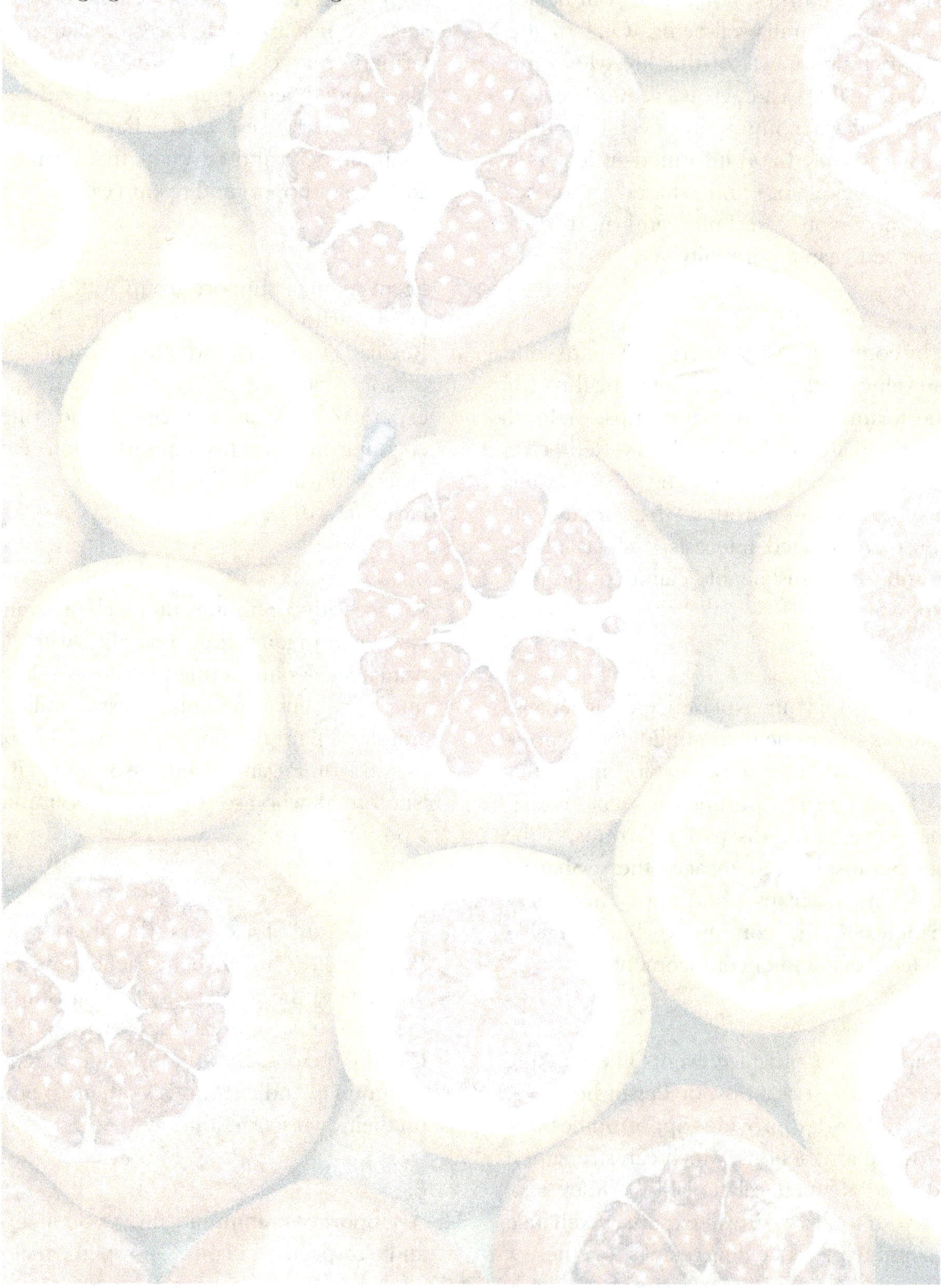

Embracing the Pegan lifestyle doesn't mean you have to sacrifice your sense of adventure or your love for dining out. Whether you're jet-setting across the globe or simply exploring local eateries, it's entirely possible to stick to Pegan principles while on the move. Here's how to navigate travel and dining out without losing sight of your Pegan goals.

1. Plan Ahead and Prepare

Before you embark on your journey, take a little time to plan ahead. Research your destination to find out where Pegan-friendly options might be. Many cities now boast a variety of health-conscious eateries that align with Pegan principles. Apps and websites dedicated to finding restaurants with specific dietary options can be invaluable tools. For road trips, pack a cooler with Pegan snacks such as fresh fruits, nuts, and pre-made salads to keep you satisfied until you find a suitable dining spot.

2. Communicate Your Needs

When dining out, communication is key. Don't hesitate to speak with the restaurant staff about your dietary preferences. Most restaurants are willing to accommodate special requests. You can ask for modifications to menu items—such as substituting grains with extra vegetables or requesting a dish to be cooked without added sugars or oils. Remember to approach the conversation with a positive attitude, which often encourages staff to be more accommodating.

3. Choose Wisely from Menus

Navigating a restaurant menu with Peganism in mind can be a fun challenge. Start by looking for dishes that are rich in vegetables, lean proteins, and healthy fats. Salads, grilled meats, and veggie-based dishes are often good choices. Opt for dishes with simple ingredients, avoiding those with heavy sauces or processed components. Don't be afraid to ask for dressings and sauces on the side so you can control the amount used.

4. Embrace Local Flavors

Traveling provides a unique opportunity to explore new ingredients and flavors. Embrace local produce and culinary traditions that align with Pegan principles. For instance, if you're in a region known for its fresh seafood, you might enjoy a grilled fish with a side of local vegetables. Similarly, local farmers' markets can be a goldmine for fresh, Pegan-friendly foods. This approach not only supports local economies but also enriches your travel experience with new tastes.

5. Make Use of Technology

There are numerous apps designed to assist with finding Pegan-friendly dining options and grocery stores. Apps like HappyCow, Yelp, and Google Maps allow you to search for restaurants based on dietary preferences and reviews. Additionally, social media platforms can offer real-time recommendations from fellow travelers and locals who share similar dietary goals.

6. Adapt Your Eating Habits

If you find yourself in a situation where Pegan options are limited, get creative. Focus on building a meal from available components: a vegetable side, a serving of protein, and perhaps a fresh salad. Sometimes, simplicity is key, and you might find that sticking to the basics works just as well. In a pinch, many places offer vegetable-based soups, grilled meats, or salads that can be tailored to fit Pegan guidelines.

7. Stay Hydrated and Mindful

Traveling can sometimes disrupt your usual routine, so it's essential to stay hydrated and mindful of your body's needs. Drink plenty of water and listen to your hunger cues. Being aware of how different foods make you feel can help you make better choices and maintain your Pegan lifestyle even when on the go.

8. Reflect and Adjust

After your trip, take some time to reflect on what worked well and what could be improved for next time. This reflection will help you refine your approach and make your future travel experiences even more enjoyable and aligned with your Pegan values.

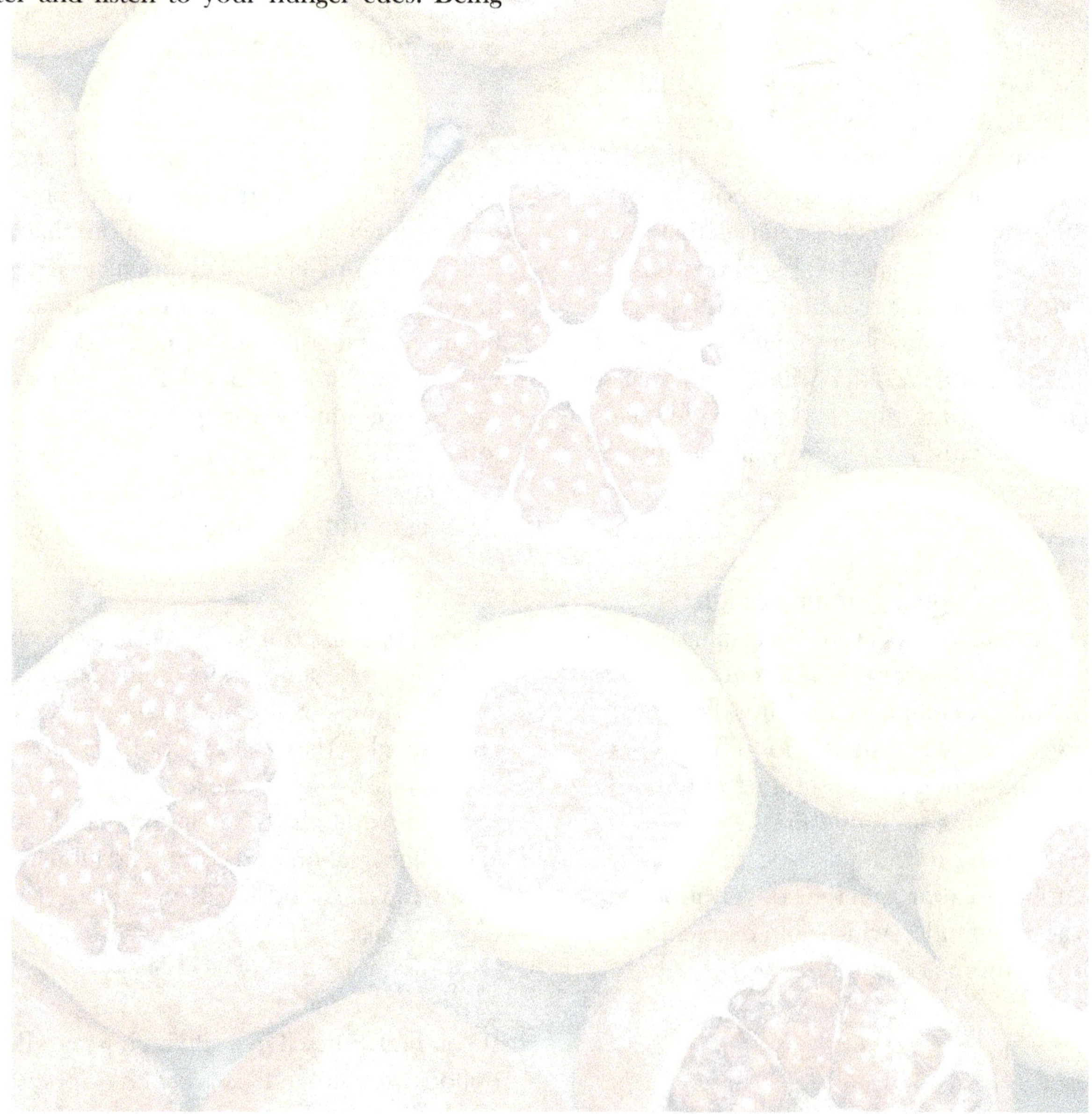

Embarking on a Pegan diet journey means embracing a vibrant, nutrient-rich way of eating that combines the best of both paleo and vegan principles. To set yourself up for success, a well-stocked pantry and fridge are essential. Here's a thoughtfully curated Pegan grocery shopping list to guide you through your weekly shopping, ensuring you have everything you need for delicious and healthful meals.

Fresh Produce

- **Vegetables:** Spinach, kale, broccoli, asparagus, bell peppers, zucchini, sweet potatoes, cauliflower, carrots
- **Fruits:** Apples, berries (strawberries, blueberries, raspberries), bananas, avocados, lemons, limes, oranges, mangoes
- **Herbs:** Cilantro, parsley, basil, mint, rosemary
- **Proteins**
- **Animal Proteins:** Free-range chicken breasts, grass-fed beef, wild-caught salmon
- **Plant-Based Proteins:** Tofu, tempeh, chickpeas, lentils, black beans, quinoa

Nuts and Seeds

- **Nuts:** Almonds, walnuts, cashews
- **Seeds:** Chia seeds, flaxseeds, pumpkin seeds, sunflower seeds

Grains and Pseudograins

- **Grains:** Brown rice, wild rice
- **Pseudograins:** Quinoa, amaranth, buckwheat

Dairy and Dairy Alternatives

- **Dairy Alternatives:** Almond milk, coconut milk, cashew milk, unsweetened coconut yogurt
- **Greek Yogurt:** For occasional use if tolerated, choose plain and unsweetened

Healthy Fats

- **Oils:** Extra virgin olive oil, coconut oil, avocado oil
- **Nut Butters:** Almond butter, cashew butter
- **Spices and Seasonings**
- **Spices:** Turmeric, cumin, paprika, cinnamon, black pepper, garlic powder
- **Seasonings:** Sea salt, tamari (gluten-free soy sauce), apple cider vinegar, balsamic vinegar

Miscellaneous

- **Sweeteners:** Raw honey, pure maple syrup (used sparingly)
- **Condiments:** Mustard, salsa (check for added sugars)
- **Snacks:** Seaweed snacks, unsweetened dried fruits
- **Frozen Foods**
- **Fruits:** Frozen berries, mango chunks (for smoothies)
- **Vegetables:** Frozen spinach, broccoli florets

Pantry Essentials

- **Canned Goods:** Coconut milk, tomatoes (for sauces and soups)
- **Baking Ingredients:** Almond flour, coconut flour (for occasional baking)

Organic and Local: Whenever possible, choose organic and locally sourced produce to reduce exposure to pesticides and support sustainability.

Read Labels: Always check ingredient lists to avoid added sugars, refined oils, and artificial additives.

Buy in Bulk: Purchase grains, nuts, and seeds in bulk to save money and reduce packaging waste

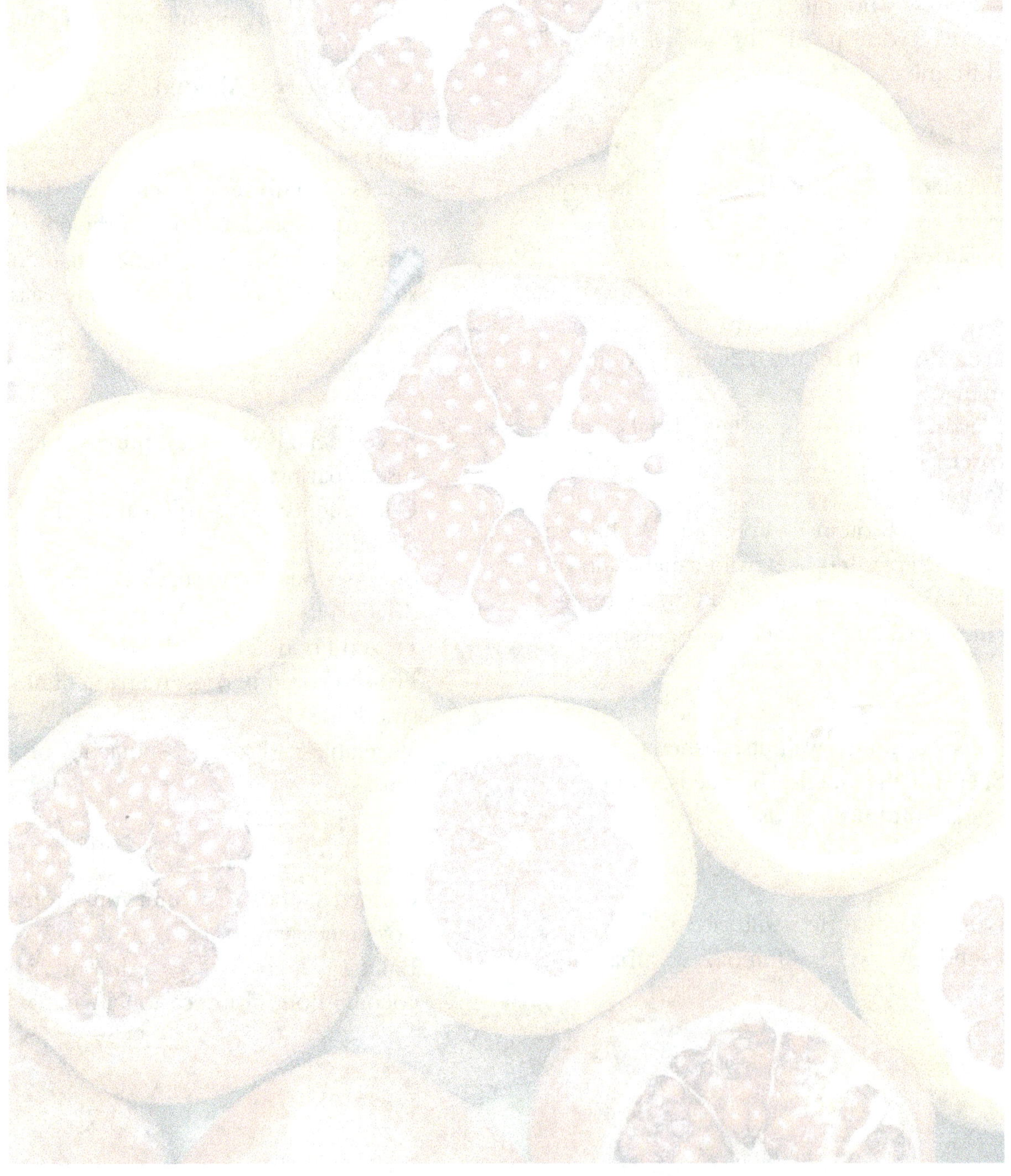

- **Almond Flour**: A fine powder made from ground almonds, often used as a gluten-free alternative to wheat flour in baking. It's rich in protein and healthy fats, adding a nutty flavor to dishes.

- **Balsamic Vinegar**: A dark, aromatic vinegar made from grape must. It's aged for a sweet, tangy flavor and is often used in salad dressings and marinades.

- **Chia Seeds**: Tiny black seeds from the Salvia hispanica plant. They are a fantastic source of omega-3 fatty acids, fiber, and protein, commonly used in puddings and smoothies.

- **Collagen**: A protein found in connective tissues of animals. Collagen supplements are popular for supporting skin elasticity and joint health, and are often included in Pegan diets for added protein.

- **Dairy-Free Yogurt**: Yogurt made from plant-based milks like almond, coconut, or soy. It offers a creamy texture without dairy, suitable for those with lactose intolerance or following a Pegan diet.

- **Grass-Fed**: Refers to animals that are fed a diet consisting primarily of grass, rather than grains. Grass-fed meat is richer in omega-3 fatty acids and antioxidants.

- **Herb-Roasted**: Cooking technique where herbs are used to season and flavor meat or vegetables before roasting. This method enhances the natural flavors while adding a healthy touch.

- **Marinara Sauce**: A tomato-based sauce typically used in Italian cuisine. It often includes ingredients like garlic, onions, and herbs, providing a savory and tangy flavor.

- **Nutritional Yeast**: A deactivated yeast that has a cheesy, umami flavor. It's often used as a seasoning or cheese substitute in vegan cooking and is rich in B vitamins.

- **Pegan Diet**: A dietary approach that combines principles from both paleo and vegan diets. It emphasizes whole, unprocessed foods, with a focus on plant-based ingredients while incorporating some high-quality animal proteins.

- **Quinoa**: A high-protein, gluten-free seed that cooks like a grain. It's rich in essential amino acids and makes a versatile base for salads, bowls, and sides.

- **Spaghetti Squash**: A type of squash with flesh that separates into strands resembling spaghetti when cooked. It's a low-carb alternative to pasta and works well in a variety of dishes.

- **Tahini**: A paste made from ground sesame seeds. It has a nutty flavor and creamy texture, commonly used in dressings, sauces, and as a base for hummus.

- ❖ Tempeh: A fermented soybean product with a firm texture and nutty flavor. It's a protein-rich meat alternative that's excellent for stir-fries and salads.

- ❖ Tofu: A soy-based protein that's versatile in cooking. It comes in various textures, from soft to extra firm, and can absorb flavors well, making it a popular meat substitute.

- ❖ Vegan: A dietary and lifestyle choice that excludes all animal products, including meat, dairy, and eggs. The Pegan diet incorporates vegan principles but allows for some high-quality animal products.

- ❖ Whole Foods: Foods that are minimally processed and free from artificial additives. This includes fresh fruits, vegetables, nuts, seeds, and lean proteins, emphasizing natural and nutrient-dense options.

- ❖ Zesty: A term used to describe foods with a bright, tangy, or spicy flavor. It often refers to dishes that have a lively and bold taste profile.

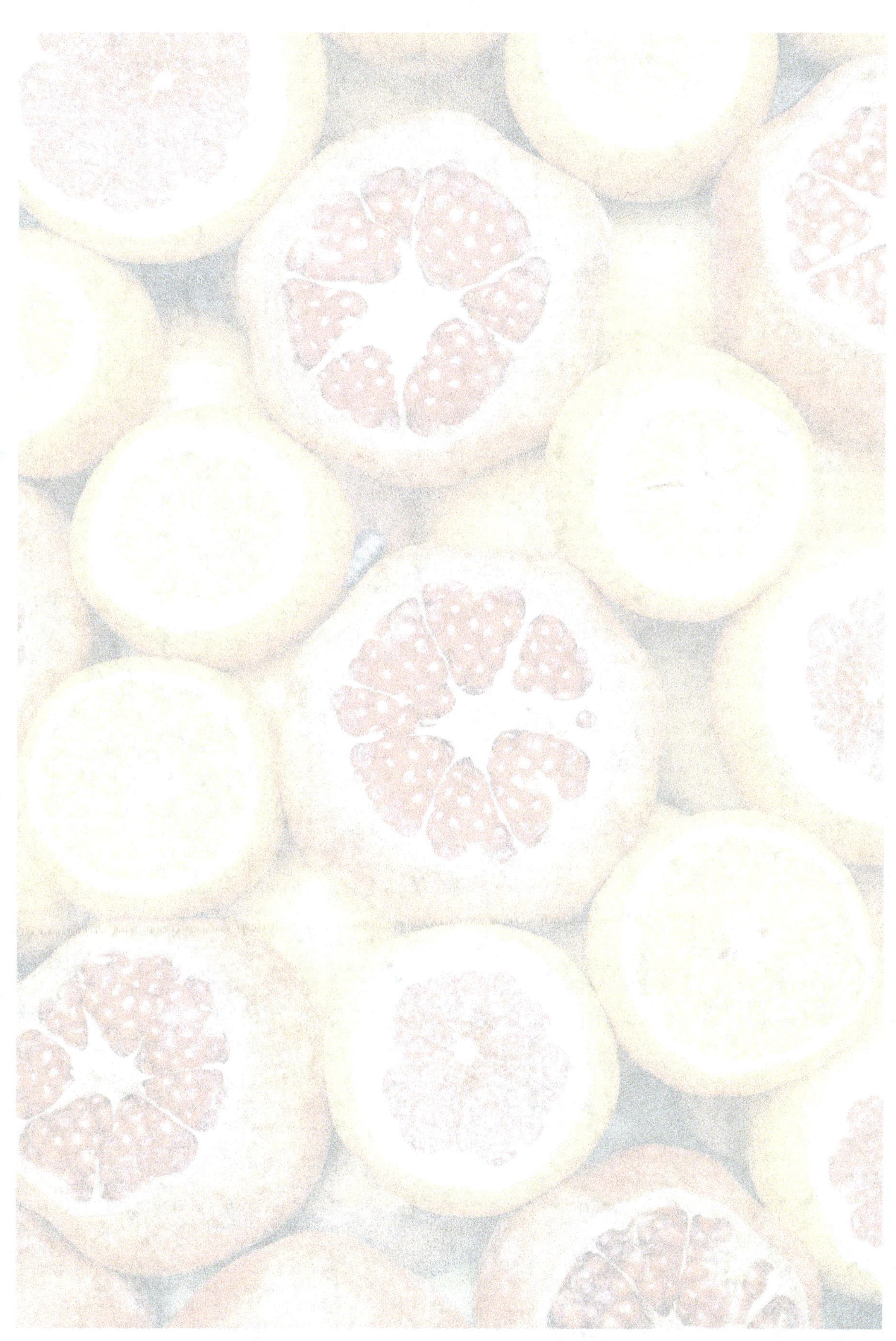